CANCER ISN'T ALL ABOUT CHEMO

CANCER ISN'T ALL ABOUT CHEMO

KEEPING YOUR BODY STRONG WHILST TRYING TO TREAT AND PREVENT DISEASE

SARAH CRIPPS

authors
AND CO.

First published in Great Britain in 2025
by Authors & Co.
www.authorsandco.pub

ISBN 978-1-917623-01-8 (paperback)
ISBN 978-1-917623-02-5 (hardback)

Medical Disclaimer

This book contains general information about medications and treatments. The information is not advice, and should not be treated as such. Do not substitute this information for the medical advice of physicians. The information contained in this book is based on the personal and professional experiences of the author. Always consult your doctor for yours and your family's individual needs.

CONTENTS

FOREWORD

BY DR KATE JAMES

It is my privilege to write in admiration of such an extraordinary family. As a human being, mother and doctor I am truly humbled by the story of little Teddy, Sarah, his mother, Kurt, his father, and his wider family. Being his doctor has been a gift.

Teddy's is an awe-inspiring story of the tenacity of the human spirit and its capacity to endure. It is a story about the power of love, the power of family, the power of hope, faith and intention, and about how a soul family may heal, even during the most trying adversity... and, in fact, go from strength to strength. This family has taught and empowered others and helped to make the world a more informed, brighter, more hopeful place.

Almost twenty years ago I found myself in similar circumstances which I could never have imagined. The second of my children, Grace, aged thirteen months, was diagnosed with a rare form of infant leukaemia and given a middling chance of cure. After the crushing feelings of hopelessness and powerlessness subsided, a fierce protectress energy arose within me, like that of a lioness protecting her pride.

I looked into my daughter's eyes and saw an incredible strength of spirit, knowing and Grace. Her name was chosen perfectly. I looked into my husband's eyes also and felt his pain more than my own. I knew we had to do everything we could to save our daughter.

Back then, as a young mother and newly qualified doctor, I didn't fully understand the magnitude of the protectress within me. I just felt it, trusted it and followed it. With three children under five, I read and researched everything I possibly could to understand how best to holistically support Grace through her twenty-six months of chemotherapy treatment. Looking back, support, guidance and help came at every step.

Grace's medical team and NHS treatment were outstanding and her Oncologist incredibly supportive. I will always remember his wise and balanced reasoning when I asked him to appraise various supplements and dietary interventions: "Kate, I can't tell you how useful these interventions will be, but I doubt they will be harmful." His collaborative approach was a welcome green light, and we began to implement a holistic protocol alongside Grace's conventional treatment.

Grace more than earned her nickname: Amazing Grace. She went into remission quickly. Her blood count recovered quickly after her treatments. We also found she needed only very occasional blood transfusions, which was unusual during such intensive chemotherapy treatment. After Grace's dietary and supplement interventions were fully introduced, she was never once hospitalised with a neutropenic infection. Again, this was unusual for a child following such an intensive treatment protocol. (Grace received treatment protocol C, the highest dose protocol, since her condition was particularly aggressive.)

Grace's Oncologist observed her progress and said to me one day, "You ought to write about this stuff!" I never did write that book but here instead is an incredible woman who did.

As Grace's and my own journey unfolded, I learned how to dance (co-create) with the universe along the way. I was shown the power of our thoughts and actions and how we create our own universe.

I learnt how to always hold trust and faith and hope in my heart. Grace fully recovered. She gained four scholarships during her schooling and became deputy head girl in her final year. I particularly remember one school sports day when, aged eight, she outran all the boys! She is now a particularly feisty twenty-year-old.

Ever since, I have been supporting and mentoring patients in my field of practice, Integrative Medicine, specialising in Integrative Oncology. Over the last twenty years of practice, I have learnt that what we often believe is impossible, may indeed be possible. I have seen patients given a 0.1 percent chance of survival get better. I hope we always remember miracles can happen.

Cancer Isn't All About Chemo is an honest, raw and incredibly informative account of how Sarah and their golden unicorn danced together. It is a liberating read which reminds us, even in the depths of darkness, there is always light.

CHAPTER 1

THIRTEEN PERCENT PROGNOSIS TO NINETY-SEVEN PERCENT CHANCE OF SURVIVAL

My biggest hope is that you are here to try and preserve your health. However, in my heart of hearts, I know that you are most likely reading this book because you or someone you love has just joined our club and you are scared stiff.

The Cancer Club. The worst club full of the best people. I am so sorry.

Cancer. It always happens to other people's families and not yours, until it does.

Right now, your mind is probably packed full of adrenaline for the fight to save yourself or someone you love, because although cancer might be the diagnosis, over your dead body will you let it win. The answer is out there, and you are going to find it.

I know this because this was me. It wasn't my diagnosis; I think I could have handled that better. My beautiful boy was diagnosed with AML leukaemia at seventeen months old and given only a thirteen percent chance of survival. His probability of survival today stands at ninety-seven percent.

Let this book take some of the mental and physical pressure away. It will give you a decent foundation of knowledge, and you can either go further down the rabbit hole yourself or just stay here. I will share with you the rules I still live by today – and today Teddy is a thriving little boy playing with his twin and giving me grey hairs for all kinds of normal mum reasons.

You haven't time for all the waffle and the fluffy stuff. I know you feel like every waking minute counts, like you are racing against a ticking clock. You just want someone to give you a step-by-step of 'this is how I did it'.

You are under pressure, trying to process all the information, all the medical jargon being thrown at you, your body is drifting constantly between fight and flight, and you probably feel like you aren't even in your own body right now.

You want someone with their crystal ball to say, "If you do what I tell you, I promise you won't lose the person you love." You know I can't do that: it would be unkind and unfair. What I can say is that nothing I will tell you about our journey will be unsafe.

This book isn't a quick fix for a cure for cancer. It is about how to put the best into your body and take away as much of the bad stuff as possible. It is about taking control where there's space to do so. Treat the body like a racehorse. Sorry to those who hate that analogy but it's the best one my brain can come up with and in the race for time against cancer, it feels like the best fit.

You will not find conspiracy theories that the cure for cancer is hidden in an African jungle that the pharmaceutical world doesn't want you to find because it wants to make a profit. Get that idea out of your head: you don't have time for that nonsense and even if it were true, it won't help you in the here and now.

Most importantly, this book is based on the principle that everything you put into your body will either help you or it will harm you. Cancer is there to harm so we need to do everything we can to balance the seesaw back in our favour. The human body is an incredible healing machine, which is why, when we fall, a scab forms and new skin grows. You might have a scar – and since you are now part of our club, emotional scars will form in your heart. I will help you with that too in this book, but first let's focus on the fight ahead. Everything else can wait.

I won't gatekeep anything. I have dedicated a whole chapter to a list of every resource I read and watched and another to give you a step-by-step plan of what I did with Teddy. The plan is suitable for people with all kinds of cancers or for those trying to prevent disease. You might need to make a couple of subtle tweaks to suit your circumstances.

Nothing in this book is wild. I know you will wonder, "Why aren't the doctors telling us this?" Please understand that they can't. They aren't deliberately hiding something that could help you or the person you love but their hands are tied. That doesn't mean my strategy isn't based on basic science, logic and common sense, it's just because that's not the way it's done.

I don't think the 'cure to cancer' out there is being hidden for financial gain, at least not by our doctors. Personally, I don't know how they do the job, especially those treating children. What pressure and what a burden. I bet they all go home and have a really good cry on the bad days and celebrate hard when another makes it to that survivor status. This book isn't here to beat up the medical system or Western medicine, but I will say that policies and procedures get in their way. Just as a boss can dictate what you do and don't say in a meeting, the medical system is the same.

However, I am a mum who got the leading cancer hospital in the UK to cook for her child to her own recipes and who openly told the medical team every single supplement her child was taking and got them agreed. I know the rules, I understand the language and I know what to say to help you get some of your own way in your mission to take back some control over cancer.

I once heard a great quote: "To follow science blindly is not science, it's religion." Science challenges thinking and explores ways to do things differently.

Certain life events stay with you forever, good and bad. You remember every sound made, every word said and every feeling in your body. There are several of these when you join the cancer club, and one particular night gave me one of mine, the night I found my missing jigsaw piece, and everything started to change. I discovered that science was actually on my side. There *were* things I could do to give Teddy a better chance at surviving cancer.

The room is dark and I'm lying on what feels like a bed of concrete. The only light is some blurry numbers on Ted's monitor, showing a nice steady, relaxed heartbeat, hopefully the sign of a good night's sleep. Everything is quiet even in the hall. It's time to do what I always do when the lights go down. More research. I need more ideas: there must be more; what if I've missed something? I can't stop now. Ted depends on me. My body is exhausted, my eyes are burning but my head is wide awake. I'll do another hour or two and that way I'll get four hours sleep and that will be enough. It's not me who needs the sleep.

It's YouTube tonight, which has served me well so far. So here we go, let's see what it suggests today. The more you watch on YouTube, the more suggestions it gives you based on what you have watched. I'm looking for the good stuff, not some crazy woo-woo nonsense saying, "Drink this weird and wonderful herb found deep in the African jungle in a tea every day and pray to this god and you will cure cancer in thirty days." I have watched sensible content and so I get back sensible suggestions.

I might be desperate to save my son but I'm also neither naive nor stupid.

And then it comes: Dr Will Bulsiewicz on a podcast discussing the microbiome with Rick Roll. Don't ask me why I click on it. I haven't heard of either of them. The podcast title isn't about cancer, but it is gut microbiome, my favourite subject.

In 2015 I started a dog wellness and nutrition brand called Frank and Jellys. I studied nutrition and helped desperate owners improve their dogs' health by focusing on their gut microbiome and diet. This podcast episode feels like something to pass the time.

I lie there half listening to their intros and a book plug. I'm not ready to give up on this episode just yet. Let's see what this 'proper' gut doctor has to say. If there's something new, I can learn from him, even if it just helps my four-legged nutrition clients, it will be worth it.

The hook comes less than five minutes in. He suddenly says, "I'm blown away by what's happening in cancer research."

I'm listening now. Sitting up. Doing that nervous tic thing where I untie and retie my hair when I'm nervous or excited. What new study? I really need to hear this.

Dr Bulsiewicz is talking about diversity within an ecosystem as a measure of health, whether that's a coral reef or the human gut microbiome (gut health). In my head I say, "Yes, yes, I know this. I've said this so many times before." That was already a pretty good win. I thought he would just give me a few great nuggets I could throw back at the doctors and dieticians next time they tried the whole, "Calories are king, it doesn't really matter what you eat," nonsense.

I could never ever have predicted what he says next. I physically jump out of bed straight into the path of our nurse for the night, Simone, very nearly sending her flying off her feet.

Eight minutes and thirty-five seconds into this interview, he utters the words, "In acute myeloid leukaemia." What the actual hell? That's Teddy's cancer. My entire body starts to tingle, my nose twitches in the way I know means the tears are coming next. I have this feeling that what he is about to say will be very powerful.

"In acute myeloid leukaemia, one of the treatments they give people is a stem cell transplant."

Check. I am sitting here two weeks post cell day. Come on, hurry up. Spit it out!

"It's basically throwing a *Hail Mary* to save a person's life. If you have a high diversity in your gut microbiome and then receive the stem cell transplant your chance of survival is actually better."

"What the…" I shout as I jump out of the bed into Simone. (Her name changed for her privacy.)

My whole body is shaking and I'm crying.

Obviously, she asks me if I'm ok. I tell her between sobs that she needs to listen to this interview from a real doctor confirming what I have always said and everything I have always fought for since Teddy was diagnosed. I rewind the video. A sense of complete relief, accompanied by anger, rushes over me. What if I had listened to them all at the beginning? What if I hadn't insisted Teddy would eat only recipes, I gave them to cook, not hospital food? Where would we be now?

At this moment, I decide that if we get through this – because it is still a big damn *if* – I am going to tell everyone who will listen. I will write a book and teach everyone how you can support the body going through cancer and it doesn't have to be hard or woo-woo or weird. It is just basic common sense and logic. And here you are reading this very book.

It probably helps that I'm not a scientist. I'm a total optimist and yet I question everything. I have a pretty good bullshit detector, so I pick at everything like a scab till it hurts and until I really understand what it means. Every waking minute not spent caring for Ted was spent researching on my phone. Secretly, I looked forward to every nap time because it gave me time to find more ideas on how to help him. This book comprises over two years of my research – everything I learned, written as if explaining it to my best friend.

That said, most of what I did for Ted is backed by science. Not all of it, to be really honest, because scientific studies take years and millions of spend and are usually reserved for big pharma who have the money to prove their drugs are safe. As an example, there aren't a huge number of studies on the benefits of turkey tail mushrooms on breast cancer and other solid tumours, but I'm pretty sure there must be a damn good reason why many Asian countries prescribe it to their patients alongside conventional drugs and chemo. But these are countries where traditional Chinese medicine – which is part of what I practised with Ted – has been part of their cultural norm for generations. Let's not forget that TCM dates back over two thousand years and that our modern medicine started with a bunch of people playing with plants.

Don't worry if people don't believe that you can contribute to a better outcome. My own husband didn't believe in my approach. It almost cost me my marriage. Now he is my biggest supporter and reminds Ted's medical team how much of Ted's success is down to what I did.

The Hippocratic oath our doctors take not to harm is named for Hippocrates, the father of modern medicine… who also said that 'all disease starts in the gut'. My hope is that you take this book to your (or your loved one's) oncologist and that they work with you as a team.

As a mother who could have lost her child and who wanted nothing more than someone to show her a better, more natural way with potentially improved outcomes, I hope this book gives *you* hope in the darkest of times because when someone we love is at risk of being ripped away from us, we need hope just to get us through the day.

Remember Simone? She took some of my book's home that night to read between shifts. Our team told me off the record that they knew what I had done and more importantly what it had done to support Ted's survival. I've met so many other parents who have adopted my methods with great outcomes. I just pray this will also be the case with yours, but you need to start now.

The nurses and health care professionals who looked after Teddy still talk about him years later. One even told another mum who found me online that in the twelve years they had worked on that ward they had never seen a child go through treatment and transplant like Teddy. He was the golden unicorn. We need more golden unicorns in this world so they can just become the norm, like horses.

CHAPTER 2

CAN WE CONTROL THE CAUSE OF CANCER?

"Your genes hold the gun, but your environment pulls the trigger."

- Dr Jack Shonkoff

Since as early as the 1920s scientists have been trying to answer one of the most important questions about one of the biggest risks to our human existence: What causes us to get cancer?

With one in two people predicted to be diagnosed with cancer in their lifetime and with billions donated every year to cancer charities, why do we still not know what causes cancer and how we can cure it?

I won't claim to have the answer to that question but I do want to share with you some interesting theories that I discovered when I was researching strategies in an attempt to save my son's life. For me, relying on conventional medicine alone and information a doctor would share with me simply wasn't enough. I wouldn't risk losing my child based upon the decisions of someone I knew nothing about. I don't want it to seem that I didn't trust our oncologist team to make the right decisions for Teddy. I didn't trust *anybody* except *myself.*

Whether it was rational or not, as his mother I felt to blame for the fact he was diagnosed with leukaemia at only seventeen months old. I had failed him, and my body had failed him whilst I was creating him. This was my fault, not his, and I had to put it right. The only way I felt I could put my head on my pillow every night in good conscience was to contribute to the solution and his survival.

I know that every parent of a child with cancer will have this gut-wrenching feeling of misplaced guilt. I know many adults diagnosed with cancer blame themselves and believe their life choices contributed to their diagnosis. If you feel this way, I want to let you know it's ok to have this feeling, you won't feel this way forever and there are better ways to channel your energy and resources. I hope this book will guide you to do this.

Thankfully, I no longer feel that guilt. I also no longer live in fear based on a narrative that getting cancer is just luck of the draw. Science has said that in fact only five percent of cancers are hereditary and out of your control. Whilst there is no doubt that genes play a role in our risk of developing cancer, I believe we have much more power over our genetics than most people would have you believe. I will also share with you the events that I have hypothesised could have led to Teddy being diagnosed with cancer.

These theories fundamentally underpin the principles of this book, the information I want to share with you and the advice I want to offer. Whilst I can't and would never attempt to claim the strategies, I used for Teddy would definitely stop you or someone you love getting cancer, dying from cancer or relapsing, I promise they will give you something pretty powerful: the feeling of control of your health and the possibility that you could influence your own destiny.

Let's look first at epigenetics and the age-old question of nature versus nurture. We all know that twins, especially identical twins, have fascinated scientists for as long as clinical research studies have been around. Twin studies provide researchers with the opportunity to test the physical and mental impact our environments have on us in an unbiased way.

EPIGENETICS

Epigenetics is the study of how lifestyle and environmental factors can affect the way our genes work without changing our actual DNA. Imagine a set of light switches that can turn our genes on or off, influencing everything from our health to how our bodies respond to stress and diet. This is called gene expression, and it can be turned on to have either a positive or a negative effect. For example, things like diet, exercise, and exposure to chemicals and toxins can lead to changes in our gene expression, which can impact our overall health and even the risk of developing diseases like cancer. So, whilst our genes might hold a blueprint for our bodies, epigenetics help decide how that blueprint is used.

In the early 2000s, Dr Robert Waterland and Dr Randy Jirtle led a now famous study of agouti mice which provided compelling evidence of the power of epigenetics. Agouti mice carry a gene which makes their fur yellow and makes them prone to obesity and diabetes. This made them great subjects to investigate the impact of the environment on gene expression.

The doctors separated pregnant agouti mice into two groups. One group was fed a standard mouse diet and the other a diet rich in nutrients known as methyl donors which are also known for their effect on brain development and function. These nutrients included choline, folate, methionine and vitamins B6 and B9.

These methyl donors help a process called DNA methylation to happen. DNA methylation is when tiny chemical tags called methyl groups are added to our DNA. When these methyl groups attach to certain parts of the DNA, they can 'switch off' specific genes, stopping those genes from working. So, having enough methyl donors can directly affect whether genes are turned on or off, influencing how our bodies function.

The outcome of the study was that the mice born from the group with the supplemented diet had darker coloured coats and a healthier body weight. This indicated that the dietary changes had led to a positive change to the gene expression of the agouti gene. In doing so it provided evidence of the potentially positive impacts of epigenetics.

This highlights not only the benefits of a healthy diet for an individual but also the potential benefits across generations. It has paved the way for many more studies into epigenetics and their influences on the development and treatment of cancer.

CANCER AS A METABOLIC DISEASE

Dr Thomas Seyfried, a researcher and professor of biology, genetics and biochemistry, has brought forward a theory that cancer is not a genetic disease but a metabolic disease.

In 2012 he published a groundbreaking book, *Cancer as a Metabolic Disease: On the Origin, Management, and Prevention of Cancer*.

A metabolic disease is a condition whereby our bodies do not use energy to process nutrients in the right way. Dr Seyfried says that it's a staged, chronic process which certainly raises questions for me as the parent of a child who was very young when diagnosed with cancer. I can't see how a child could get a chronic condition unless it's been passed down from the mother.

However, I have also read about the large volume of heavy metals identified in recent years in the umbilical cords of newborns, obviously passed from the mother. Maybe it is time that science revisits the true impact of a mother's diet and lifestyle in pregnancy and what this could mean for predicting a child's future health based on what happens when they are in the womb.

You might wonder how that research made me feel – it could suggest that I could have done better to help avoid Teddy's diagnosis. My intention is not at any point to make anyone feel blame or shame, but I feel a duty to share with you what the science says to give you the full picture so you can formulate educated opinions, and so we can all try to do better in the future.

Do I blame myself, based on Dr Seyfried's theory? Do I think I could have played a part in the diagnosis? Actually, I don't. No one can blame themselves for not knowing what they don't know. I did my best as an expectant mother with the advice given to me by healthcare professionals. If I were looking for someone to blame, I would blame the food industry and its hiding of nasty health-damaging ingredients in plain sight, slowly causing silent issues every time we put food in our mouths. All in the name of profit for shareholders. I would also blame our modern society that makes us all believe that unless we run ourselves into the ground trying to do it all, we aren't contributing enough to the world. It isn't socially acceptable to put yourself and your health first. It's a great mission statement for employers and governments but in my opinion, in practice it's simply lip service.

There is strong evidence that cancer cells behave differently from healthy cells in terms of how they get energy. I touch on this a little more in Chapter 8 on complementary therapies, in which I talk about the Warburg effect.

It has been claimed that cancer cells prefer to produce energy in a way that is less efficient than healthy cells. Instead of using oxygen to break down sugar fully, they do it in a way that creates waste products like lactic acid. This method helps cancer cells grow and divide quickly, which is why they can become difficult to control.

Additionally, the tiny structures in our cells called the mitochondria, which are like mini factories, don't work as they should in cancer cells. These mitochondria usually help our cells produce energy and also trigger cells to die when needed – when cells are damaged, for example. But cancer cells find ways to keep growing and avoid this self-destruct feature.

Thinking of cancer as a metabolic issue highlights the importance of our diet and lifestyle choices in reducing our cancer risk. For example, diets high in sugar and unhealthy fats (which I call fake fats) may encourage the faster energy production we see in cancer cells.

On the flip side, eating whole foods like fruits, vegetables, healthy fats and proteins can help keep our metabolism working well and might even lower the chances of developing cancer. Some people are looking into low-carb diets, like the ketogenic diet, which could potentially help slow cancer growth by changing how the body processes energy. The keto diet has been supported by many outspoken doctors of functional medicine and integrative oncologists, especially for cancer patients with solid tumours.

Dr Seyfried and his colleagues have spoken passionately about the use of ketogenic diets in helping reduce tumour sizes in glioblastoma to allow surgical removal to take place. Glioblastoma to date is one of the deadliest cancers with really poor survival rates and which does not respond well to radiation therapy – the current standard treatment plan. The doctor says it is key to lower blood sugar and elevate ketones for all cancers and to supplement the diet with glutamine-targeting drugs to attack the tumours.

Exercise also plays a big role in cancer prevention in terms of our metabolism. Regular exercise or sport helps our metabolism stay healthy, reduces inflammation and boosts our immune system. This can also reduce our risk of getting cancer. Maintaining a healthy weight can also support a reduced risk.

When you look at this in combination with epigenetics, there is a lot of strong research and evidence to highlight a connection between how our bodies process energy and how our genes behave. Changes in metabolism can affect the nutrients available that help modify how our genes function. Byproducts of energy production and metabolism have the potential to send signals that influence gene behaviour, potentially leading to cancer growth.

THE 'DIRTY GENES' CONCEPT

The phrase 'dirty genes', introduced by Dr Ben Lynch, describes specific genetic variations or changes that can disrupt how our bodies typically work, especially concerning metabolism, detoxification and overall wellbeing. Having researched his work for some time, I feel that the concept of 'dirty genes' relates to what I have learned about epigenetics and cancer as a metabolic disease using genetics *and* ties into some of the more traditional scientific views that cancer is caused by your genes.

In his book, *Dirty Genes,* Dr Lynch highlights how these variations can trigger a range of health problems, including a higher risk of conditions like cancer. He stresses that understanding how these genes work is essential for us to grasp the complex relationship between our genetics and the environment around us.

When we talk about 'dirty genes', we're not saying they're fundamentally broken or bad. Instead, we're referring to genes that don't perform at their best due to mutations or small changes, known as single nucleotide polymorphisms (SNPs). These variations can weaken the body's ability to detoxify harmful substances, process nutrients from food properly and handle stress. All of these are crucial for keeping your body strong, staying healthy and preventing disease.

Dr Ben Lynch talks about seven key genes that are really important when it comes to our health and the risk of diseases like cancer. Knowing how these genes work can help us understand how our genetics, along with our environment and lifestyle choices, can influence our health. Due to the growing interest in Dr Lynch's work and people's desire to understand how their bodies' gene expressions work, you can now order at-home methylation tests online. Labs can try to identify your gene variations so you can look to make lifestyle changes to optimise your health.

SEVEN KEY GENES AND THEIR ROLE IN THE RISK OF CANCER

1. MTHFR (Methylenetetrahydrofolate Reductase)

This gene helps the body process folate, a crucial B vitamin for making and repairing DNA. Variants in the MTHFR gene can disrupt folate use, leading to increased homocysteine levels, an amino acid linked to a higher risk of heart disease and certain cancers. Those with MTHFR changes might benefit from eating folate-rich foods or taking supplements.

2. COMT (Catechol-O-Methyltransferase)

The COMT gene produces an enzyme that breaks down hormones like dopamine and oestrogens. Variants can impair this process, throwing off hormone balance and increasing the risk of hormone-related cancers, such as breast and prostate cancer. Understanding this gene can help people make better lifestyle and dietary choices for hormone health.

3. DAO (Diamine Oxidase)

This gene breaks down histamine, a compound involved in allergies and inflammation. If DAO isn't working properly, it can lead to high histamine levels, causing allergic reactions and chronic inflammation, which could be linked to cancer. Knowing about the DAO gene can help individuals avoid high-histamine foods, potentially lowering cancer risk.

4. CBS (Cystathionine Beta-Synthase)

The CBS gene processes sulphur and helps detoxify harmful substances. Variants can disrupt sulphur metabolism, leading to higher levels of homocysteine and other harmful compounds. Elevated homocysteine can cause oxidative stress and inflammation, both of which may promote the development of cancer. Eating the right foods can support healthy sulphur metabolism and reduce these risks.

5. SHMT (Serine Hydroxymethyltransferase)

This gene is vital for one-carbon metabolism, crucial for DNA synthesis and repair. Variants can affect the availability of necessary substances for healthy DNA function, potentially leading to genomic instability, which can increase cancer risk. Consuming foods rich in folate and other B vitamins can support the SHMT gene and help lower cancer risk.

6. AGT (Angiotensinogen)

The AGT gene helps regulate blood pressure and inflammation. Variants may disrupt levels of angiotensin, a hormone that manages blood pressure. If this control is off, it can lead to increased blood pressure and inflammation, both of which are linked to cancer. Maintaining a healthy lifestyle with regular exercise and a balanced diet can help keep blood pressure in check and reduce cancer risk.

7. MTRR (Methionine Synthase Reductase)

The MTRR gene is key for managing homocysteine levels and supporting DNA methylation, a process that regulates how genes express themselves. Variants can disrupt this balance, leading to elevated homocysteine and issues with DNA repair, which can stress cells and heighten cancer risk. Ensuring adequate intake of nutrients like folate and B12 can help this gene function properly and lower the chances of developing cancer.

For the longest time, I wrestled with wanting to understand the cause of Teddy's diagnosis and why it was Teddy who got leukaemia and not George. Not because I would wish it on either child of mine but here was a confusing example of nature versus nurture and its influences on health. Teddy and George are non-identical twins. Their birth weights were very similar, both were born by elective caesarean, and both were raised in the exact same way eating the exact same foods.

One reason I was hell-bent on trying to understand this was because I was terrified for George and his risks of getting leukaemia in the future.

My cousin Michael, a first cousin on my father's side, died from leukaemia when I was eleven. He was only twenty-two. I felt that I had passed on this bad gene of mine, which added to my feeling of guilt. That being said, I have always been led to believe that a family history of disease carries more significance on the maternal side. My cousin Michael was my dad's brother's son. Also, my dad's brother doesn't have the same father as my dad. So, from a genetic perspective, it seems more of an unlucky coincidence… but then again, if you could see Teddy and George against my husband Kurt and me, Teddy looks just like me and George is just like Kurt. Maybe Teddy carries more of my DNA than Kurt's.

I felt that if I could understand why Teddy became ill and not George, I could do more to try and prevent a cancer recurrence or it impacting more members of my family. But our hospital didn't seem concerned about George's risk levels when Teddy was diagnosed and when we identified that Teddy needed a bone marrow transplant to save his life, we tested George, hoping he could be his donor. We found out that George was not a close enough genetic match. You could argue that this in itself reduces George's risk, but I feel there was more to it. I think it all started with our first family holiday.

When the boys were eleven months old, we took them to a five-star resort in Greece, a well-known brand favoured by parents of young children. I mean, this place was so child friendly they would be brushing away the food fight that had landed on the floor as soon as it occurred without batting an eyelid. Whilst we were at that resort the boys picked up a hideous stomach bug or food poisoning. It was violent and vile. I have never seen a child projectile vomit so much and so frequently. I thought we were going to end up in hospital with the boys.

George was so sick the first evening that by the end he was vomiting yellow bile. It seemed like he really had got a lot of it out of his system, and he felt better a few days later. Teddy wasn't as sick as George on that first night, but it lingered for so much longer and his immune system seemed to take a knock in the few months after the holiday.

That was in September. By the end of November or early December, Teddy had caught RSV (actually three RSV strains) and spent a week in hospital on oxygen therapy only to come out of hospital to catch Covid-19 ten days later. A few weeks after he had recovered from Covid, we started seeing signs of what appeared to be a viral infection such as a runny nose, without any clear causes. He ended up with two lumps on the back of his head that concerned me, so I took him to the GP and thereafter for a second opinion, which led to his diagnosis of AML Leukaemia.

Hippocrates, known as the father of medicine, is famous for saying that all disease starts in the gut. From my work and studies, I know the power of gut health and the immune system. It could be that the damage done to Teddy's gut health at the time of our holiday started the ball rolling, causing inflammation and a leaky gut. Leaky gut, also known as dysbiosis, is a condition by which there is an unhealthy level of bad bacteria in the gut. These bad bacteria can damage parts of the intestinal wall called villi and microvilli and even create small holes in your intestines which result in food and pathogens leaking into your bloodstream. This can lead to high levels of inflammation in the body which can go on to cause autoimmune conditions or other chronic diseases because the body is not able to absorb nutrients adequately.

Considering the theories of epigenetics, dirty genes and cancer as a metabolic disease, I can logically place the holiday incident as that first step in the damage of Teddy's immune system and the subsequent illnesses he struggled to fight off, resulting in the development of his cancer. Whilst I can't currently tell you about the dirty gene variations Teddy holds, I plan to test for them. Not just for Teddy but for all my family. Knowledge is power: the more we know, the better choices we have for ourselves and our individual needs. With this, we can lower our risks of disease.

Whilst I may not have known about all the scientific theories on the causes of cancer when I started my journey to getting Teddy back to health, I discovered them along the way. They only validated our strategies further and motivated my family to continue.

The theories of epigenetics and cancer as a metabolic disease are highly suggestive to me as reasons why some people with an extensive family history of cancer never go on to develop cancer themselves, and why we hear of people with a terminal diagnosis going on to have a spontaneous remission following radical lifestyle changes. They take away some of the arguments from sceptics that diet and nutrition have no influence or role to play in the prevention and treatment of cancer and other chronic diseases. The more we understand our own unique dirty genes, the more we can tailor our diets and lifestyles to maintain control not only over cancer as a society through epigenetics but over other chronic diseases that affect the quality of life for millions of people all over the world.

CHAPTER 3

DIET AND NUTRITION

"Let food be thy medicine and let thy medicine be thy food."

- Hippocrates, father of medicine

This has been the hardest chapter for me to write. The information is not difficult to explain or complicated to understand and replicate; it's actually super simple and backed by research and thousands of years of history. It has been hard because I want to put across everything I know about diet and nutrition passionately enough for you to become deeply invested without making you feel judged or pressured.

I have learned through personal experience over the last ten years that the conversation about what you feed yourself, your child or your pet is probably as divisive as politics and religion – maybe more so. I fully understand the challenges you could be going through. Whilst the chemo was being pumped through Teddy's veins and not mine, I lived and breathed it as if it was treatment for my own disease.

Before sharing the specifics about diet and nutrition, I would like to answer some of the big questions you probably have about nutrition and oncology. A common question is, "If what you eat can affect your oncology journey, why don't doctors tell us what to eat during treatment?"

Firstly, doctors don't receive nutrition training so they can't. During a four-year undergraduate degree, medical students only receive twenty to thirty hours nutrition training, and there's no evidence of further nutrition training thereafter. On average, it takes eleven years to become a doctor, including the training they require to reach their specialism.

Secondly, there is not the formal clinical research to back up any medical advice regarding the food a patient should eat. Without proven studies, doctors won't make recommendations. Reputable research takes many years and several hundred thousand pounds at a minimum. The funding source is either governmental, the pharmaceutical industry, or academic/not-for-profit groups. The profit-making industry has the most amount of money at their disposal, but they are disinclined to fund research into the benefits of broccoli sprouts as an anticancer agent, for example. There is no profit nor an ability to trademark or patent a food.

This is not a wild conspiracy theory. Just look up one of the world's leading cancer hospitals in the US that tried and failed to patent broccoli sprouts as an anti-cancer agent. It is public record. We have to consider what will generate a return on investment for these multi-billion-pound companies. There is simply no value in investing all that money in something people can grow on their kitchen windowsill in less than five days.

My nutrition journey started in 2015, running my online supplement and wellness business for dogs. I knew how divisive the topic of nutrition was even then when talking about dogs, let alone someone navigating cancer treatment. But when one of my dogs started struggling with yeast issues (candida) which resulted in ugly stains on her face and bad skin, I decided to go all in when someone offered me an opportunity to learn more about gut health. I have never looked back. I was able to help desperate dog owners make huge improvements in a short period of time with nutrition plans. Some of these dogs had been on seriously strong medication for prolonged periods of time with no success. One was even facing the threat of being euthanised. This was why I felt an inner voice telling me not to discount the power of nutrition when Teddy was diagnosed.

I had some of the skills and the understanding based on mammals as a whole, but I needed to go in deep and quickly. In my head, like yours I expect, I heard a ticking clock, and I was running out of time. Every second had to be used for the right purpose.

I want to stress again that I am sharing my journey and everything I have learned so that you could potentially live a healthier life or support someone going through cancer treatment so that they can hopefully have the same experience as my son had. I in no way judge anyone who doesn't want to take the same approach. It is not for everyone. In the past, I was sometimes so fearful of being ostracised by my own oncology community that I said very little and kept my knowledge to myself. But if I can help one more adult or child have a similar experience as Teddy, of course it is worth a bucketful of criticism and trolling.

When Teddy was diagnosed, just as we were coming out of the pandemic, I was your pretty average sleep-deprived first-time mum with twins, struggling through the days and trying to do a good job. I had set my personal goal early on that I didn't want to be cooking two different meals every evening. Having grown up in a house where my mother was an incredible cook and all our meals were made from scratch, I was drawn to cooking from a young age. In my adult relationships I showed love through home-cooked meals. It was my love language. That being said, yes, my children had eaten fishfingers and I did allow a biscuit or two, but they had a healthy diet on the whole and I encouraged healthy eating as part of our weaning journey, even if it meant using shop bought pouches.

Would we eat the way we do now if Teddy hadn't been diagnosed with cancer? I highly doubt it, although not for want of trying. I lacked and still lack what ninety-five percent of the modern world lacks: time. There is an expectation that mums will raise children like they don't work and work like they don't have children.

The experience of many oncology children, past and present, compared with Teddy's experience was like night and day. This is not just in my opinion but in the opinion of every single medic who was part of Teddy's wider oncology team. Teddy experienced no major side effects as a result of treatment, and he didn't even lose his hair till after his bone marrow transplant. No painful mouth sores (mucositis) that stop people eating, no need for pain medication, he never stopped eating after we started our supplement and diet regime, and he required no synthetic milk or intravenous feeds.

This is absolutely unheard of. Our senior transplant consultant had to back pedal when she returned from three weeks' leave after the donor cells were infused into Teddy's body for transplant, sheepishly telling me in a quiet tone, "I stand corrected; I got it wrong about nutrition. I have always been interested in the gut microbiome."

It should have felt like a huge victory, as one by one doctors and nurses shared their admiration of Ted's success. It didn't, because I know they had been sniggering behind our backs before they had to stop when he didn't get sick, unlike the others. I know from one of our favourite nurses that it was the hot topic of conversation in the staff room. They started paying attention and asking questions. As my mum always said to me as a child, "The one who laughs last, laughs loudest."

But cancer is no laughing matter, ever. I'm lucky – my child is here despite a horrendous prognosis. I just wish a doctor would ask me in detail about the strategies I implemented and looked at the science was behind it. It is just food, which can't harm. The hospital cooked for Teddy from my recipes so the nutritional differences he was having compared to the other children were no secret. I wasn't paying for them to do so, and many other parents requested some of my recipe from our hospital, especially a nutrient-dense vegetable broth that appeared to do wonders for many of them in terms of warding offside effects of treatment during transplant. It is a real shame that nobody has asked me yet as I believe many could experience remarkable benefits.

You did read that right. I convinced the leading UK cancer hospital to cook to my recipes for my son because their food was garbage. I am not interested in bashing the medical system but when a single bag of chemotherapy with a significant acceptable failure rate costs £20,000 (as told to me by a healthcare professional), in my opinion, you should strive to do better than serve overcooked vegetables (which removes all the nutrients) with a sea of beige ultra-processed garbage that no one in their right mind would encourage even a healthy child to eat.

I attempted to make the right noises by engaging with the head of the hospital kitchen. I intend to do more of this in the future. Unfortunately, in order to make a difference, I need the doctors to make the first grumbles and then for the decision makers to sit up and pay attention – especially because the right diet can save money in medications prescribed for side effects. In the oncology world, you have your chemo, then a drug for the side effects and then another drug for the side effects of the drug for the side effects. I kid you not.

Dr John McDougall, an American doctor, is famous for saying, "Everything you eat will either help you or harm you." Largely, I subscribe to this statement. Facts are that when we eat unhealthy foods, ultra-processed foods or foods that have been altered so that a company can have them last longer and make more profit, the body has to remove what is not a natural substance that it can use and excrete it. This puts extra work on some of the vital organs like the liver to remove stabilisers, preservatives and emulsifiers.

In my opinion, when your body is going through oncology treatment, it needs the most TLC and support and the least stress possible. In this instance, reducing stress means trying to reduce the time it spends processing food that doesn't serve it so it can do what's most important, which is help eradicate cancerous cells alongside the use of conventional medicine.

So, let's take you on a journey of the art of the possible if you fuel your body in a healthy way… backed by research. You will find links to credible resources in the further reading chapter.

Here is a crash course in gut health and the gut microbiome. I am thrilled to see that in my two and a half years thus far in the oncology community so much more information about the importance of the gut microbiome is coming into the mainstream as a result of the incredible work of people such as Dr Will Bulsiewicz and Tim Spector.

Approximately eighty percent of the immune system sits in the gut. The first time I ever said that to a medical doctor back in 2022, I remember them arguing, 'black was white', that this was incorrect. These days, they are a little less defensive based on people with authority telling them it is so and not a crazy oncology mum on a mission to save her son's life and have input to his treatment plan.

The gut microbiome is a collection of trillions of microscopic organisms that sit in your gut and digestive tract, mainly your large intestine. They are largely made up of bacteria, fungi and viruses. Some are harmful if they go unchecked and can lead to things like yeast, but for the most part they are super helpful to the body and its functions. They even impact the brain and its functions due to something called the gut-brain axis. Think of them as an army of workers who take what you bring into the body and try to turn it into something useful that the body needs. This helps balance your hormones and mood, supports your immune system and your digestive system, and even manages inflammation and regulates your blood pressure.

The microbes that make up your gut microbiome need different foods to keep themselves alive and to replicate when an individual microbe comes to its natural end of life. This is why we need a huge variety in our diet and why we should act with caution when it comes to antibiotics. Antibiotics wipe out good bacteria as well as the bad and if you do not have a healthy and diverse diet, some of those helpful microbes could be lost forever. This can be true even if you have never used antibiotics but just have a poor diet. It can take up to a year for the body to recover its lost helpful bacteria after some types of antibiotics.

When we were in transplant there were so many rules to keep Teddy protected from infections. We had to be isolated as much as possible and Teddy was not allowed to leave his room for several weeks, so we bought a brand-new fridge and asked the hospital for permission to have it in our room. This allowed us to reduce the time spent in the ward's family kitchen where another parent might be carrying a virus without symptoms. Someone from the estates team came to check it out and then my husband and I were able to nourish our bodies to the best of our abilities by eating pre-cooked fish or chicken with salad and fermented vegetables like kimchi.

This kept our gut microbiome happy and in turn, it helped us stay as mentally strong as we could. When I was surviving on fizzy drinks, sandwiches and snacks, I felt like my anxiety was constantly through the roof. I was living very much on a knife edge. Being mindful where I could about what I was eating really helped my general anxiety levels both during Teddy's treatment and post-transplant.

However, I recognise that not always knowing what to eat for the best can lead to feelings of overwhelm. If grabbing a sandwich and a bag of crisps or a pasta salad is all you can manage based on the setting you find yourself in, that's ok. Control the controllable where you can.

Genes play a part in our health and our risk factors for acute and chronic diseases. Although we cannot control the genes we were born with, we can influence our microbiome quickly and for the better so that we have the upper hand when it comes to epigenetics and reducing the risk of a life-changing diagnosis.

This is why I become irate when I hear people say, both inside and outside the oncology world, that calories are king, and it doesn't matter what you eat. It absolutely does matter. If you have a low budget to feed your family or you have a picky eater in your home, I acknowledge that it could be hard. It is hard. But so is cancer. You just have to decide if it is important to you and, if it is, get creative.

If you are struggling you can always reach out via my website **www.cancerisntallaboutchemo.com** for resources and support, whether you are in treatment or not. I have become the queen of hiding the healthy stuff. I regularly share recipes via social media channels to help you hide more diversity in your diet, so it doesn't feel like such a chore. Let's be honest, there are only so many salads anyone wants to eat and so many fights you want to have with your family to get them to eat them. I understand all the challenges of picky eating that come as a result of taste changes during conventional treatment.

Many people experience taste changes as a side effect of chemo. When I surveyed people in a social media group right back at the beginning of Ted's treatment, all those who said they had been personally affected said that food often tasted like cardboard. The conventional advice tells you to eat bland foods. I suggest doing the opposite: eat food full of flavour. We didn't go crazy making our foods really spicy, but we experimented with herbs to give food and its flavour real depth. Garlic and onion, ginger, miso and turmeric were some of Ted's favourites during treatment.

Probiotics and probiotic foods were a no-no during treatment. Probiotics are not recommended on the basis that they have 'live' bacteria in them and are a risk to an immune system that's been compromised by chemo and radiation. Prebiotics were allowed, however, so we focused on prebiotic foods and supplements. Prebiotics are the food for the good bacteria that's already in your gut system. They include things like onion, garlic, chicory root, asparagus, bananas, apples, lentils, chickpeas, nuts and seeds to name just a few. Please note, you want to aim for a variety of these in your diet.

Reflecting on everything I have learned; I think there is probably more value in focusing on prebiotics than probiotics. My theory comes from this. You might not know which bacteria your gut is lacking if you haven't carried out a stool sample test. You could literally be throwing money down the toilet by using a probiotic supplement as the body gets rid of what it does not need. The body knows what it needs the most. By focusing on a wide range of prebiotic foods, you provide food for all the types of bacteria and let your body decide which it needs to replenish.

In the days following Teddy's diagnosis, I also stumbled across the work of Dr William Li, a world-renowned medical scientist with a biochemistry degree from Harvard who leads the Angiogenesis Foundation. The moment I saw his TED talk "Can we eat to starve cancer?" I felt like all my blessings had come at once, just when I needed them, backed by the world's best nutritional scientist (in my opinion).

If food and lifestyle medicine is a subject of interest to you, I encourage you to read some of Dr Li's books. I will link to these in the further reading chapter.

In summary of what is probably his most famous piece of work, Dr Li's talk focuses on blood vessels, how they play a role in the formation of cancer and autoimmune conditions, and how certain foods can potentially support the regulation of those blood vessels. This is called angiogenesis.

The TED talk helps us understand why blood vessels are so important to the body. We are given our bodies' required number of blood vessels in the womb. They are part of the healing process when we fall and cut our knee. The blood vessels self-regulate their number and size based on the body's need. In the event of an injury, they grow under a scab to allow the wound to recover and then prune themselves back to the right length based on the body's own inhibitors of angiogenesis.

The body's blood vessels have a set limit to their growth and don't grow further or decrease unless the body's angiogenesis is out of balance. When levels of angiogenesis are too high it can result in diseases such as cancer, psoriasis, endometriosis and Alzheimer's, to name a few. When levels are too low it can lead to conditions such as neuropathies, pre-eclampsia, stroke and chronic wounds. According to Dr Li, approximately seventy diseases affecting many people across the world have ties to imbalances of angiogenesis.

You might wonder why I am writing about this, given Teddy had blood cancer. Apparently, excessive angiogenesis is a distinguishing aspect of cancer – all types of cancer. There I was with a glass of wine in the dark in my bed, pausing the TED talk constantly, rewinding it and taking notes and more notes so I could build a meal plan focused on anti-angiogenesis foods. The strategy was to cut off the food supply to the cancerous cells. I can't cover all the details here, but I highly recommend further research into Dr Li's work, in particular his TED talk, which is less than twenty minutes long.

I know what you really want is the list of foods that made it onto our meal plan. There are others which you can uncover with research, but this is a high-level list of foods I felt I could get into Teddy's diet.

TED'S ANTI-ANGIOGENETIC FOOD LIST

Strawberries	Blackberries
Raspberries	Red grapes
Apples	Pineapple
Cherries	Oranges
Maitake mushrooms	Kale
Pak Choi	Garlic
Turmeric	Ginseng
Parsley	Soybeans
Pumpkin	Tomato
Tuna (wild caught)	Lemon
Dark chocolate	Whole grain rye
Green tea	Lentils
Kidney beans	Artichokes
Walnuts	Almonds
Pistachios	Flax seed
Chia seeds	Pumpkin seeds

If you follow Teddy's social media pages, you may note from the recipes I share that these foods still form a big part of Teddy's diet today despite the fact we are no longer fighting cancer. This experience has changed our lives, and we are deeply invested in keeping our family as healthy as we are able to and can afford to.

In summary, here are some of the principles of the diet plan that I put in place for Teddy based on what you have read above. You can find further details and some taster recipes in Teddy's step-by-step plan in Chapter 11.

My strategy was to give Teddy a diet high in fibre from as many different plants as possible, including fruits, vegetables, beans, nuts and legumes.

Thirty-five to fifty different plants in a week are a good target. When you write it down and get creative, you will see it's not as hard as you might think. Also, you can work with me, and I will help you.

One approach to reaching the food diversity goal is to base your eating on the commonly known concept of 'eating the rainbow'. Foods of different colours are said to have different benefits for the body.

Foods that are naturally red in colour like tomatoes, strawberries and bell peppers are high in antioxidants like lycopene and anthocyanins, which may support healthy skin, a healthy heart and even reduce the risk of certain cancers. They also tend to be high in vitamin C which is good for the immune system.

Orange and yellow foods like carrot and sweet potato are often rich in substances like beta-carotene which the body converts into vitamin A. These are good for your immune system, your eyes and may help in reducing inflammation and oxidative stress.

Green foods such as leafy greens, avocados and green beans are packed full of vitamins such as A, C and K. They are usually high in fibre and antioxidants, which support your digestive system and reduce the risk of chronic diseases. Some even contain chlorophyll which supports the body's natural detoxification process.

Blue and purple foods (blackberries, aubergine, red cabbage, etc.) are rich in anthocyanins which also have antioxidant properties that have been linked to improved brain health and a reduced risk of certain diseases. They may also lower inflammation and improve cognitive function so are a great addition to the diet of children with developing brains.

White and brown foods like garlic, bananas, cauliflower and mushrooms might not be super colourful but don't let that fool you. They can be full of great nutrients like potassium, fibre and antioxidants. They may help support a healthy immune system and your digestive system. In addition, onions and garlic are full of allicin which has a ton of health benefits.

I appreciate that there is a huge amount of information here about nutrition. Just try your best to get as much as possible of the good stuff into the body rather than focusing on removing the bad. Tools like the slow cooker, even in warmer months, were a lifesaver for me when I was trying to get everything done with such a busy diary. You will be surprised how quickly taste buds adapt and change and cravings for processed and ultra-processed food naturally subside. You may even find what you enjoyed before unpalatable.

If you feel deeply invested in changing your diet but are not sure how to implement it because you spend long periods of time in hospital, I am here to help you via my website. Later chapters will also help you make the first step in the direction.

CHAPTER 4

SUPPLEMENTS

"A good supplement is nature's gift
to help you achieve your best self."

- Unknown

So, what is a supplement? It can mean different things for different people, but the official definition is a product that provides additional nutrients that could be missing from a person's diet that have the potential to improve their health and wellbeing.

I will tell you about different types of supplements in this chapter, what to look out for, and why I think some are better than others.

Had this book landed in my lap when Teddy was diagnosed with leukaemia, I know this is the first chapter I would have gone to. I couldn't have waited. When you have a ticking time bomb in your head, you look desperately for a pill, a powder, a capsule – albeit a natural one – that could blow cancer or the risk of cancer into the abyss never to be seen or heard from again. Some research suggests that up to sixty percent of cancer patients upon diagnosis may search online for the 'best supplements for cancer patients. I think we are all looking for a quick fix to make life perfect, some of us just more urgently than others. If that's you I totally understand.

Our supplement journey started when Teddy was less than a month into his diagnosis, carried out under the watchful eye of the UK's leading cancer hospital. I was only ever fully transparent and honest with them about the supplements I gave Teddy.

Whilst they tried to discourage me by telling me they didn't recommend supplements, I quickly learned that even though Teddy was part of a clinical drug trial this did not mean we were not allowed. I have dedicated a whole chapter to the words *"we do not recommend"* and suggest you visit that chapter next if you don't intend to read this book in order, before you do further research and discuss your intentions with the oncology department treating your or your loved one if you are in active treatment. You can also read the chapter which details Teddy's step-by-step plan that my family and I implemented during and after treatment, which includes the supplements we used.

It might surprise you, if you have read the previous chapter on nutrition, that I recommend taking supplements. I truly believe that most of the world should be taking supplements in one form or another, whether they have been impacted by cancer or not. The food industry has changed, and the quality of our soil has been eroded due to pressures on farming practices and the invention of the modern supermarket.

I haven't gone all conspiracy theorist on you. For farmers all over the world to keep up with the demands of mass food production, the quality of our food has suffered and with it have some of the nutritional benefits we gain from eating the produce. For example, a blackberry purchased from a supermarket doesn't carry anywhere near the same punch as it did if you went blackberry picking twenty or thirty years ago, although even today they still taste very different if you stumble across a wild blackberry bush out on a walk and pick one to eat.

Minerals are amongst the nutrients that have been most depleted in our bodies due to food mass production. Magnesium, zinc, iron, calcium and selenium have all been scientifically documented as in decline in people due to how the soil is taken care of and the heavy use of chemical fertilisers. These essential minerals are key for our immune system and our overall health. Magnesium, for example, is responsible for approximately three hundred different processes in the body. It is key in turning food into energy, it supports our bones, helps regulate blood pressure and is vital in the growth of new healthy cells. It is also a key component in our mood thereby supporting our mental health.

The other biggest cause of depleted magnesium within the body is *stress*. Between the decrease in the nutritional value of food and the pressures of modern life, we are already pretty screwed.

It is estimated that four out of five people are deficient in magnesium so it's now one of my favourites for all my family. In an ideal world, of course I recommend you look to explore proper testing to see which nutrients you are deficient in before spending money on supplements. However, I recognise that this can be expensive, and you may not be motivated to do so, so I will tell you what I can about supplements and what to look out for.

Whilst conventional chemo, radiation and immunotherapy have the intention of saving a person's life, they also damage the body and deplete it of vital nutrients. This can be due to the side effects of treatment which can result in nausea, vomiting and loss of appetite or a common but more serious side effect called mucositis. All of these affect the volume of food some people can eat or impact the desire to eat nutrient-rich foods.

In addition, the drugs themselves can damage gut health and the gut microbiome, disrupting the absorption and metabolism of nutrients. This can lead to a condition called dysbiosis (leaky gut) which is incredibly difficult to diagnose and a multitude of longer-term chronic health issues including autoimmune diseases as a result of increased inflammation. According to scientific research, some of the most common nutrient deficiencies cancer patients face include a deficiency in protein, iron, vitamins (such as vitamin D, B12 and folate) and minerals (such as magnesium and potassium).

Hospitals rarely test for some of these deficiencies and for some not at all. Interestingly, doctors seem the least resistant to cancer patients taking vitamin D supplements, given many of them take it themselves. Vitamin D is mainly absorbed through the sun's natural rays on bare skin. If you are a cancer patient who is avoiding the sun at all costs or spending long periods in hospital without sunlight exposure, vitamin D supplementation will potentially be beneficial. My personal suggestion is to seek out a vitamin D3 and K2 supplement.

Vitamin D3 also helps the body absorb calcium from the diet, which is important for our bones. K2 ensures the calcium is directed to the bones and not the soft tissues and arteries, reducing the risk of cardiovascular diseases.

Even though my family has been out of the treatment process for a while, we all still take vitamin D in the autumn and winter months as we live in the UK where it gets dark quickly and it rains a lot.

In spring (when it's warm enough) and in summer I encourage the children out in the sun in as little clothing as possible from as early as seven am until the UV rays become unsafe. Many people are unaware that vitamin D cannot be obtained from the sun if you are wearing sunscreen. Try to get your bare skin in the sun when it is safe to do so. Even when Teddy was spending time in hospital as an inpatient, we would walk him in his buggy to a beautiful hospital garden so he could get some natural vitamin D every day. Vitamin D has been said to play a significant role in immune health and especially respiratory health. Some research points to links between Covid-19 and vitamin D levels in an individual person, affecting their mortality risk.

I was a little ahead of the game in understanding the benefits of supplements due to my online canine supplement business. I didn't just want to take Teddy's body back to its baseline whilst he went through treatment. I wanted to do more and help his body eradicate this mutation that was causing havoc and threatening his life.

I knew that if anyone out there in the UK could provide me with a reputable professional to support Teddy using natural methods, they would be in my community. I was already in the natural and holistic industry and had connections to some of the best people, who in turn had access to the best people I hadn't heard of. To this end, I made a choice to go public on my personal social media and tell the world that Teddy had leukaemia approximately two weeks after he was diagnosed, and the initial shock had worn off.

Enter Dr Kate James. My inbox flooded with well wishes, amongst them a recommendation that I contact Kate. I can't now even remember who that person was, despite having searched my inbox to thank her. She helped save Teddy's life, even offering to give up her own appointment if it meant getting into Kate's fully booked diary. Dr Kate, as we call her at home, is a traditionally trained doctor and is still on the General Medical Council's register. Her daughter had leukaemia as a toddler almost twenty years ago and is now a beautiful, thriving university student. It was a match made in heaven.

I remember desperately emailing her, begging for an online appointment. Her out-of-office reply said that she was on Easter holidays with her family but gave a mobile number and I felt I couldn't wait for her return. I texted her to plead our case as I had been advised her patient list was full.

She agreed to meet with me, and while it was an agonising wait, I felt a sense of calm. Help was on the way. In the meantime, I just focused on keeping Teddy's diet clean by adding in the good stuff and trying not to put myself under pressure if my husband Kurt allowed him to eat the occasional naughty snack.

Some doctors might have a level of ego about their work that you should just accept everything they tell you at face value. But that's not the type of Doctor Kate is. What I love about Kate and her approach is that she doesn't hold back on giving access to any of her academic contacts to ask more questions about research and studies.

If you or someone you love is in active treatment for cancer, I highly recommend you try to work on a one-to-one basis with a naturopathic doctor or an integrative doctor or practitioner with a science and medical background where possible. You want to work with someone who has authority and credibility and understands basic blood work. I wish more such people were available, although I can see a huge increase in people coming into this field.

I was ready to start supplements with Teddy the second I met with Dr Kate, but being the incredible doctor she is, she slowed me down just a little. She wanted to know all the medications Teddy was taking, and the results of his latest blood work and bone marrow biopsy before putting a plan together. Whilst emotionally we all just want to chuck the kitchen sink at cancer, we have to be strategic and support the body, not burden it by making it get rid of things it doesn't need.

The number one natural supplement I feel in my heart of hearts as an oncology mum that every cancer patient should have prescribed to them is IP6 and Inositol. If you do nothing else to preserve your health or consider in order to fight this awful disease, please look at this supplement in detail.

Without IP6 and Inositol, I can't say where I think we would be. Teddy and his twin George will take this for the rest of their lives.

IP6 and Inositol, also known as inositol hexaphosphate, is a naturally occurring product found in many foods, particularly high-fibre foods like grains, seeds and legumes. There has been a lot of interest in IP6 and its involvement in cancer prevention, cancer treatment and managing chemotherapy side effects since the 1990s with many academic research papers written on the topic. Professor Shamsuddin, one of the academic contacts Kate introduced me to from her little black book, pioneered the research into IP6 and cancer. He started his research into the formation of cancer back in 1975 in one of the USA's leading medical university research departments.

Neither my doctors nor I had heard of it until Kate came into our lives, even though I had done a huge amount of research into supplements before our appointment. My hospital said they didn't recommend I give it to Teddy and their reasoning caused me concern. Professor Shamsuddin was more than happy to give me information, without making any ridiculous medical claims, that helped me feel safe and reassured me this was the right supplement for Teddy with our diagnosis. In fact, reading back on old emails I can see that I was able to teach the hospital pharmacist a thing or two about how not to misinterpret studies.

At this point I feel it's important to stress again how Teddy flew through his treatment, never stopped eating and had no major side effects, including not losing his hair till after his bone marrow transplant. He took IP6 three times a day in his bottle, but it can also go down an NG tube or Peg (discussed in later chapters).

I will always remember the day Teddy took IP6 for the first time. It is one of those oncology memories ingrained in my long-term memory. I had in my haste ordered IP6 from abroad as Kate was awaiting new stock and it was late in arriving. Teddy had been admitted to our local shared care hospital due to a blood infection that could have been avoided. He was thin, his immune system was drained, and he had this huge ulcer hanging from his top lip touching his top teeth. He wasn't eating and my mental health was on the floor.

The IP6 had arrived. Kurt delivered it to me at the hospital. I gave Teddy the doses as prescribed, and the hospital said we could all go home till his next antibiotics were due in eight hours' time – we were only a five-minute drive away. So, home we went to try to perk him up by spending time with his twin.

Later that day, I looked at Teddy and the ulcer had just vanished. I thought it had burst. I checked his mouth, and it had literally gone back in on itself. I went back to the hospital an hour and a half early that night before the shift handover so our nurse, Annie (name changed for her privacy), could confirm that the ulcer had in fact deflated in a few hours. It was unbelievable. I knew if I tried to explain it to the night shift, they would think I had gone crackers, and Annie was my only witness having seen it earlier that day. I mean, this thing was huge.

That night, Teddy woke up in the hospital after a couple of hours of sleep and demanded food. I sobbed. I had been desperate for him to start eating again so I could get good nutrition into him. He ate five whole slices of toast, which was all we could get for him at that time of night. I wasn't prepared with food from home because he hadn't been eating. After that, my child never really stopped eating in active treatment other than for a short period during transplant when I wasn't allowed to give him IP6.

While so many struggle through treatment, Teddy isn't the only one who didn't. Many people around the world tell a similar story. That, plus the research that suggests that IP6 has the potential to slow down the progression of cancer cells, makes this, in my opinion, a must for all patients.

One of the most common questions I am asked via our social media is what multivitamin I recommend, generally. I have to say, I am not a fan of multivitamins for a couple of reasons. Firstly, the dose of individual vitamins in a combination product is never enough to have any real benefit. Also, in my opinion, the companies selling these usually add fillers and binders and things I wouldn't consider putting into my child's body, especially some of these chewable gummies.

Teddy was and still is far too young to swallow capsules and tablets, so I try as much as possible to get our supplements in a liquid or powdered form. I taught Teddy to accept the liquid supplements by opening his mouth like a little bird and I often hid powders in food or the bottle of oat milk he drinks twice a day. Usually, we would have been encouraged to wean him off a bottle by his age. However, it's more important that he gets those key nutrients into his diet than we worry about his teeth formation. After speaking to a close friend of mine who's one of the best dentists and maxillofacial surgeons in the country, though, she assured me that as long as Teddy doesn't use the bottle like a dummy his teeth will be fine.

You could choose to research different types of supplements outside of standard vitamins to help keep the body strong and in balance, such as minerals, amino acids, fatty acids, probiotics, enzymes and herbal supplements. Please note, however, that most oncology teams won't sign off probiotics during active treatment as they are live bacteria. We started probiotics approximately eighteen months after Teddy's bone marrow transplant, mainly because we were focused on the other types.

Below you can find a quick reference table with some examples of supplements. I have also added food sources to the table as I think we should always try to get as many nutrients as possible from food.

Supplement Type	Example of Clean Supplement	Food Sources
Vitamins	Vitamin C	Citrus fruits (oranges, lemons), strawberries, bell peppers, kiwi, elderberry
	Vitamin D3+K2	Fatty fish (salmon, mackerel), egg yolks, fortified milk
	Methylated vitamin B12	Animal products (meat, fish, dairy), fortified plant-based milks
Minerals	Magnesium	Irish sea moss, nuts (almonds, cashews), seeds (pumpkin seeds), leafy greens (spinach)
	Zinc	Irish sea moss, oysters, red meat, poultry, beans, nuts
	Iron	Red meat, lentils, beans, spinach, fortified cereals
Herbal Supplements	Turmeric (curcumin)	Turmeric root (add black pepper)
	Ginger	Fresh ginger root, ginger tea
	Broccoli sprout extract (sulforaphane)	Broccoli sprouts, Brussels sprouts, kale
	Ashwagandha	Ashwagandha root (often consumed in powder form)
	Adaptogenic mushroom powders	Reishi, cordyceps, lion's mane, chaga, turkey tail (more information below)

Supplement Type	**Example of Clean Supplement**	**Food Sources**
Amino Acids	L-Glutamine	Meat, fish, eggs, dairy products, spirulina, tofu, red cabbage, beetroot,
	L-Arginine	Meat, poultry, fish, dairy, nuts (especially walnuts), chickpeas, black beans
	L-Tyrosine	Chicken, turkey, fish, dairy products, some nuts, edamame beans, tofu
Fatty Acids	Omega 3 (e.g. DPA, EHA)	Fatty fish (salmon, sardines, mackerel), flaxseeds, chia seeds
	Omega 6	Nuts, seeds, goji berries
Probiotics	Lactobacillus (probiotic strain)	Greek yoghurt, coconut kefir, sauerkraut, kimchi, miso
	Bifidobacterium	Yoghurt, fermented dairy products, certain cheeses
Enzymes	Bromelain	Pineapple
	Papain	Papaya
	Lactase	Lactose-free dairy products, fermented dairy

Through our treatment journey and my research, I became more and more intrigued by the practices of traditional Chinese medicine (TCM) and Ayurvedic medicine which comes from India. Both practices have been around for over two thousand years and hold the objective of restoring balance within the body. Their principles vary slightly and can be adopted simultaneously, as far as I am aware, which is certainly what I did for Teddy.

My strategy and plans to keep Teddy healthy and strong leaned more towards TCM, in part due to Kate's influence, I think, as she also practised in this area. For example, when Teddy was first home after transplant and was catching winter germs, I focused on foods and recipes that supported his lungs and spleen. In TCM it is the belief that the spleen is key to the absorption of herbal medicines and food, which in turn are beneficial for overall health. As part of my further research and discussions with Kate, I learned all about adaptogenic mushrooms and I have been pretty obsessed with them ever since.

Adaptogenic (or functional) mushrooms help your body adapt to stress and support the body's overall wellbeing. This includes environmental and physical stress, not just emotional stress. They are natural substances that promote homeostasis in the body. The term *homeostasis* means *balance within the body*. Homeostasis is key to keeping us alive and managing important bodily functions such as body temperature, acidity level and the balance of salts and blood sugar levels.

You can grow many of these mushrooms at home in the right environment using specialist kits, but that felt like too much work for me at a time when I was dragging myself through the days in survival mode. Instead, I had Teddy take adaptogenic mushroom powders prescribed by Kate. You can purchase them from other providers online, but I suggest you reach out to sellers first and ask about the environments in which the mushrooms are grown.

Ideally, look for a supplier who grows their mushrooms organically, without the use of pesticides. Ask if they use the mycelium *and* the fruiting body of the mushroom. The mycelium could be described as the roots (although it is not that simple). For the best quality supplement, you want a combination of both but ideally with a higher amount of fruiting body. I also favour supplements that have been created using a double extraction method as these are more easily absorbed by the body, giving greater benefits.

Southern Asian countries have frequently prescribed adaptogenic mushrooms alongside conventional treatment for their cancer patients. The one that has attracted the most interest in the oncology world is turkey tail. Research and studies suggest that it may encourage cancerous cells to commit apoptosis (i.e. suicide) without damaging healthy cells.

I have added information below to enable your further research. Again, these are supplements we all still take at home, some of which have been invaluable to my own anxiety levels through the journey we have been on.

Reishi (Ganoderma lucidum)	"Mushroom of immortality" – Reishi is believed to support the immune system, promote relaxation, and reduce stress and anxiety. Promising studies researching the use of reishi to induce cell suicide in human leukaemia cells
Cordyceps (Cordyceps sinensis)	Potential to enhance energy, reduce fatigue and give the body a boost. Cordyceps may also support respiratory function and overall vitality. Said to be a potent anti-viral. Great for adrenal support. Promising studies using cordyceps in lung and ovarian cancer patients.
Lion's Mane (Hericium erinaceus)	Potential cognitive benefits, including support for memory, focus and nerve health. Promising studies using lion's mane for anti-tumour effects in colon cancer.
Chaga (Inonotus obliquus)	Known for its high antioxidant content. Thought to help support immune health and combat oxidative stress. Promising studies on how chaga may stop cancer cell proliferation for a wide variety of cancers including oral cancers.
Turkey Tail (Trametes versicolor)	Recognised for its immune-boosting properties and often used alongside conventional treatments in cancer support therapies. Promising studies across a variety of cancers for turkey tail's anti-tumour effects and improving quality of life for those undergoing treatment.

With regards to the use of supplements either as part of a cancer preventative health journey or a journey in active treatment, in my opinion you cannot out-supplement a poor diet. Whilst I appreciate this may feel like a huge challenge if you are spending a lot of time in hospital, there are options to make small but powerful changes. Where you can, focus on fresh whole foods. Learn to read labels. The fewer ingredients, the better, and if you can't pronounce an ingredient or recognise it as something you could have at home, avoid it.

Even without the most optimal of diets, supplements can have a huge impact on your body, in particular the immune system to keep it as strong as possible. With a clean diet, though, you can really turbocharge the benefits.

Before ordering supplements, if you aren't working with a functional medicine practitioner or integrative oncologist as I recommend, I stress that you must do your research before knee-jerking and making an impulsive purchase via Amazon. Fish oils and Irish sea moss can contain heavy metals based on the state of our oceans so ensure that you are buying products from companies that care enough to test their products for heavy metals before selling them. Don't be afraid to email the manufacturers. The supplement industry is heavily saturated with companies offering similar products: I believe it is every company's job to evidence why you should spend your money with them.

If your budget doesn't allow you to buy organic food, I would focus on organic supplements such as broccoli sprout extracts, fish oils and elderberry syrup. If in doubt, my social media accounts will also guide you to some of our favourite supplements that we use following heavy research.

CHAPTER 5

WE DO NOT RECOMMEND

"There are no facts, only interpretations."

- Friedrich Nietzsche

I encourage and in fact plead with you that however you choose to approach your oncology journey in terms of supportive therapies or supplements, you are always transparent with your medical team.

Eradicating cancer needs all hands-on deck, and you should feel that it is a partnership. While both sides may not always be on the same page about everything, a great deal can be achieved when both parties know there is an underlying foundation of transparency and respect, and everyone knows when they need to be the one to bend a little.

That being said… "We do not recommend" doesn't mean *not safe*.

Read this chapter in full before having a discussion with your team about the supplements you would like to pursue alongside and in support of your conventional treatment. I want you to read it because I want you to be in a position to make an informed decision. Ultimately, it is the patient's choice (provided it's not illegal) what supplements they want to take and everyone else is there to guide from their knowledge and experience.

However, I also know what your medical team will say, word for word, when you approach the subject of supplements. I know the seeds of doubt they will plant. More importantly, I know exactly why they say those specific words and phrases. It's not why you think.

You will sit down with the oncologist or nurse and the conversation will very likely go like this:

Patient: So, I have been doing some research and looking at the benefits of taking X, Y, Z for my type of cancer. Is that ok, can I do that?

Medical professional: We don't recommend taking supplements during treatment.

Silence.

Patient: But why? It's all natural.

Medical professional: Even though it's natural it could still interact with your medications and there's very little evidence that it can help treat cancer.

Patient: Ok, so are there any foods I should eat or foods I shouldn't eat?

Medical professional: Not really, just avoid grapefruit whilst you are on chemo and no yoghurts with live cultures. Try and eat a healthy and balanced diet but at the end of the day, as long as you eat to keep up your strength that's the most important thing.

Patient: Ok, so you are saying there is very little evidence that supplements help but you aren't saying there is no evidence they can. And in the same breath, you are telling me I can eat anything I like, yet you don't recommend the supplements I'm asking to take… which are mainly food-based products.

Does this sound familiar? Maybe you think I'm psychic. If I were, that lottery win would have been mine a long time ago. I know because it's what I was told and it's what every oncology parent I have ever met who wanted to do supplements was told. They heard the words as: "We aren't allowed."

Let's dissect this a little further. I'm channelling my younger sister into this chapter. She is a very successful lawyer who's very clever with her words and who, over the years, has taught me the importance of language and word choice.

To recommend is "to put forward (someone or something) with approval as being suitable for a particular purpose or role" (Oxford dictionary). It is the *proactive* encouragement of something. Your traditional medicine oncologist will not proactively encourage you to take a supplement that has not been individually tested against each of the medications on your treatment plan. Imagine if they did and you got really sick because you chose to take milk thistle to protect your liver alongside your chemo… or it caused your chemo not to work properly… or even worse, it caused death. Families would sue and rightly so. If someone told me something was safe and it turned out not to be, somebody's head would roll.

Then again, I also had to sign some pretty nasty consent forms against the damage that chemo could have done to Teddy and even the risk to his life of having a Hickman line inserted during surgery. In case you haven't come across a Hickman before, this is an internal line inserted from outside of the body to the heart. They pump medication and chemo through it and also use it to extract blood for regular testing.

Today we are celebrating two years of remission for Teddy. Looking back, today of all days, and thinking about something that was actively pumping poison straight into my child's heart has made me feel a bit queasy, even though that poison also saved his life. I am so proud of how far he has come, and I have zero regrets about taking our own path to get here. A big part of that was pushing back when the dietician on the team first said, "We do not recommend supplements."

What follows is an account of how it was accepted by Teddy's medical team that he would take supplements whilst going through active chemotherapy.

In Chapter 4 you read about our guardian angel, Dr Kate. She is a naturopathic doctor who helped us alongside our oncology team at the hospital. Kate originally trained under the National Health Service in the UK. Her daughter had leukaemia twenty years ago as a child similar in age to Teddy, so she knows what it's really like. One of the things I really liked about Kate was that she didn't gatekeep any of her academic contacts so that I could do full and thorough research.

Before I met Kate, I was just pulling on my experience of nutrition including how I had advised people to support a healthy liver. In the first days of being admitted to our primary care oncology hospital our dietician, Lisa, had told me that the milk thistle I wanted to give Teddy to protect his liver from the chemo was not a good option. What she probably said was that they did not recommend it… but in my mind, I heard her say that it was a 'no go'. That was my first interaction with the confusing statement: "We do not recommend". At that time, I was out of my depth, panicking and wanting to throw everything natural at Teddy's body to protect him. Thank God Kate came into our lives when she did.

I am a bit of an oversharer by nature and sometimes far too honest for my own good. Being less than honest with my team about supplements Kate had recommended didn't even cross my mind. But I was also scared. I always wanted to be responsible and seek medical advice before starting Teddy on anything. The whole thing was new territory, and I needed people around me to act as guard rails to help keep Teddy and me safe. Whilst the medical team and I didn't always agree and they often said, "We do not recommend," there was only one time they said something was unsafe. This was when I wanted to give Teddy a supplement called lucuma powder, a Peruvian superfood, and they said it would interact with a transplant medication. I didn't even question it that time. I did as I was told because we had built up what I believe was mutual respect and understanding – and above all, trust.

If you are told by your medical team that something is unsafe, you must listen. You don't have to agree with what they say, but you have to be transparent, and you have to listen to safety warnings.

After getting Dr Kate's support a month after the diagnosis, I wrote an email to my team with details of Kate and her credentials and our plan. I chased up a few times as the response wasn't as quick as I would have liked, and I was desperate to get started.

Late one afternoon, Lisa came into our room with a stack of printed papers, Memorial Sloane Kettering branding across the top of it. They are a very famous New York oncology hospital. Look up what they say about certain supplements and be sure to read the parts for health care professionals, because the difference in the narrative is often very interesting.

Lisa crouched next to my armchair and started working through each one of the supplements one by one to tell me why they weren't recommended.

I remember certain events on this journey very clearly and this is one of the clearest, because I lost it. My blood was boiling. I didn't shout because I wouldn't risk upsetting my child, but I really showed her my teeth. "Thank you for your input but given the fact that you have come back and said no to every single one of them, I'm not convinced you are acting in the best interests of my child," I said.

At this point Ted, not wanting to miss out on the drama, grabbed the papers out of my hand where he was pulled up on the side of his baby jail cot and threw them everywhere. It felt like a "Yeah take that, we aren't going to listen to you."

Thanks Ted... talk about making a situation even more awkward.

I wasn't going to be a total arsehole and leave them there; I had to clean them up.

I told her I had no intention of reading the material. I trusted Kate and I trusted myself and my extensive research. However, I promised her that I would always let them know what I was giving Teddy because whilst we didn't agree on this, for Ted's sake we had to work together. It wasn't personal, but at that moment I lost faith. I think, on reflection, had they come in with a compromise on supplements based on a risk assessment, I would have complied. I felt dismissed and even more determined to do it my way.

She was quite upset about the interaction. I apologised at a later date, not because I felt I was wrong with what I said but because my delivery could have been better. She and I later had multiple civilised disagreements during treatment, and I really gave her a run for her money given my nutrition background. However, when all was said and done, she went above and beyond for Teddy in transplant regarding nutrition and my wishes. After we were discharged, I left her a gift at reception of some of my favourite cancer nutrition books by reputable authors. I hoped that she could potentially move the needle from inside the system. After all, she had seen firsthand how Teddy responded to treatment.

Doctors do not recommend supplements simply because they can't. Their hospital policy doesn't allow them to, the pharmaceutical industry does not allow them to (by not doing safety testing of their drugs alongside common supplements and vitamins) and their personal liability insurance doesn't allow them to. That doesn't mean that natural supplements taken in moderation are unsafe. When you give a supplement that is food based, not synthetic, the body will excrete what it does not require. In fact, many South Asian countries give adaptogenic mushrooms such as turkey tail mushrooms to breast cancer patients alongside their treatment. Traditional Chinese medicine is part of their culture, not a trend.

Unfortunately, I have recently learned that the breakthroughs that happen in the lab take twenty-five years to make it down to mainstream treatment. If I waited for others to have the same opportunities as Ted, we would be talking about my grandchildren's generation. This is why I have written this book.

Doctors' hands are tied. It's not that they don't want to help. They *can* help and they *will* recommend supplementation if you have the data to back the need for it.

So how do you get the data? Chemo and radiation therapies have been evidenced as depleting some vital nutrients and vitamins such vitamin D, vitamin B12, folate (vitamin B9), magnesium, vitamin C, vitamin K and vitamin B6. I recommend asking your medical team to test your levels prior to starting treatment and regularly assess these. If you are deficient your team will be required to prescribe supplementation – although not necessarily the best versions, in my opinion. Refer back to the supplements chapter for more information on choosing the best supplement options based on vitamin requirements.

CHAPTER 6

STRESS

"Self-care is a way of taking responsibility for yourself. It means showing up for yourself like you would for someone you love."

- Brené Brown

It is really important that we talk about stress in a meaningful way, and I hope I can give you some real tools to manage your stress levels. If one more well-meaning person had told me to be kind to myself and to try and practise self-care where I could for even five minutes, I think I would have self-imploded. I needed real tools that didn't involve going for a walk or reading a book.

Navigating a cancer journey for yourself or for someone you love is like the worst roller coaster of deep depression and crippling anxiety. It is purely survival and dragging yourself through the days until (hopefully) that day you hear the words 'no evidence of disease' and can ring the end of treatment bell. Even though the journey doesn't end there, that's the goal everyone is working towards.

This chapter is about the practical things I did to get me through the times of Teddy's chemo, his bone marrow transplant and the period afterwards when we were counting down the days to the ultimate goal of two years post-transplant. I learned some of these things for myself and some of them from learned professionals whose help I asked for. I will be open and honest with you that I now suffer with PTSD since Teddy's treatment, and OCD with intrusive and worrying thoughts but not an obsessive desire to clean. My anxiety was so high at times I could do nothing but pace a room pretending to distract myself with tidying up but really achieving nothing.

Before we dive right in, I have one request to make, and I make it only to help this journey be marginally easier. Whether you are going through cancer treatment yourself, or supporting someone going through treatment, please let your network of family and friends help you. They want to help. You cannot do all this by yourself. It takes a village, they say, to raise a child and you need the whole damn town in this fight against cancer. Delegate the things you can so you can focus your energy into fighting this disease. Let people help you.

It is not just because of your mental wellbeing that I want to help reduce your stress. It is also for your physical health, because as the medical field will tell you, stress is the silent killer.

When you are under stress your autonomic nervous system will put your body into one of three modes. You have probably heard about them before: flight, fight or freeze. During this time, the body releases two commonly talked about hormones: cortisone and adrenaline. Cortisol is a key part of your body's stress response and helps regulate a number of key functions including the metabolism and the immune system. It can be helpful in the short term, providing energy and focus should you ever be chased by a bear in the woods, but in the long term it can be hugely detrimental to your health. This probably explains why I dropped so much weight before my wedding day without ever going on a diet and why I have gained over three stone (19kg) since we hit the one-year post-transplant mark despite having a pretty great diet on the whole. Chronic stress, which is part of our journey to survivorship, can have a serious impact on your physical wellbeing, not just your looks.

On a cellular level, high levels of cortisol and chronic stress can disrupt the process of healthy cell creation and repair, which could slow down the healing process for oncology patients. By that, I mean damaged tissues and organs. It can weaken your immune system and its ability to function, which again is key for repairing damaged cells. With a weakened immune system, you are more susceptible to getting sick. Whether you are the patient or the caregiver, this isn't the time for recurring infections and germs.

It can also increase oxidative stress within the body. In lay terms, it's like having too many bullies in the school playground (free radicals) and not enough superheroes (antioxidants). The bullies can cause real damage to your cells and whereas normally the superheroes would come in, clean up the mess and save the day, there simply aren't enough of them. Oxidative stress has strong links to cancer.

I say all of this not to fear monger or to suggest that if you feel stressed you will automatically get cancer or impact the outcome of an already diagnosed cancer, but to stress (pun intended) that this is not the time to be a martyr and try to handle everything by yourself. It will lead to an over-boiling pot and an even greater mess to clean up afterwards.

I speak from firsthand experience on this, and that's with the help I had.

My husband's favourite phrase to say to me is and was, "Sarah, you need to stop trying to control everything and control only the controllable." He began saying it after Teddy's diagnosis and still regularly says it to me even now, just about things in life. And he's right, but there are a lot of things you do have control over during a cancer journey provided you have a committed support system around you, which I really pray that you do.

Let's talk first about friends and family. When I made the decision to go public with Teddy's diagnosis in order to find a good naturopathic doctor, the floodgates opened with messages from friends and family, some of whom I hadn't heard from in years. They wanted to share their sadness for our family and offer their help, hope and best wishes, but it also meant more people who wanted to know how he was doing and have regular updates on his treatment.

Some people in the oncology world opt to have public social media accounts where they can push out a message and an update just once and everyone can see it. Some opt for private groups either on social media or a private messaging app. We did a bit of both, but I had clear rules for myself and for others.

Whilst I totally understood that close family and friends who loved Teddy were emotional about the diagnosis, I had a strict rule that people couldn't cry in front of me. If they did, I would pass the phone over to my husband or find an excuse to close down the call early. I couldn't handle being responsible for someone else's feelings when I was fighting for my son's life. Also, I made it clear that if I wasn't posting on social media, it was because there was nothing to tell or he was feeling pretty rotten, so people shouldn't chase me directly. I tried to post at least once every four days to avoid direct messages, and I kept all my notifications off so I wouldn't be disturbed unless it was on my terms.

As much as I didn't want to do it, my dogs went to stay with my parents who lived a couple of hours away. I don't think I asked for it, but my dad drove down in that first week when we knew Teddy wasn't coming home soon and insisted, he take some of the added pressure off our plate. Otherwise, I would have struggled through as my dogs were like my first children. Unfortunately, my youngest dog Lulu passed away whilst she was in my parents care from a cancer no one knew she had. In one of those weird coincidences, she passed in the same fifteen minutes as the doctors came in to tell us Ted's transplant had been a success. I felt so guilty that I hadn't been with her, but I know she will forgive me. It feels like she gave up her life so he could have his.

Ask for help to care for your pets, whether you have someone take them or you get a spare key cut to care for them on a pre-agreed schedule. Perhaps you feel guilty asking for help or that you should be able to do it all – that you should be strong enough and capable enough. I want you to know that it is totally normal to feel this way, but neither is true. Please do not struggle. We all have the same hours in a day and, unfortunately, cancer has decided for you that it's going to consume your every waking moment. It's not fair but then, cancer isn't fair either.

My sister was a key force in helping me navigate this journey and became a second mum to Teddy's twin, George. She and I are only two years apart and whilst we fought like cat and dog growing up (even now, sometimes) she was an incredible support to me during Ted's treatment. The day he was formally diagnosed she drove up to the hospital, alcohol stashed in her handbag and told me if there was ever an appropriate time to drink alcohol in a hospital it was the day your eighteen-month-old was diagnosed with cancer. For the record, she had four alcohol drinks with included mixers – and no, I didn't drink them all.

She immediately set up a WhatsApp group for herself, my mum, Kurt's mum and Kurt's sister. They were there, ready and waiting, to coordinate care for George so we could reduce the impact on him as much as possible. Having a key point of contact person who is a 'doer' who can coordinate other people's actions will give people a sense of purpose and contribution and will also be a lifeline for you. She also took George on as many fun activities as possible that she was already doing with my niece Holly who's a similar age to George and Teddy. Kurt and I are both truly grateful for the way she and her husband Harry just accepted George as a surrogate child into their weekend plans.

My in-laws were also incredible and took George abroad on holiday for a week. The idea of him being in another country without me tore me up inside, but it was what was best for him. I completely recognise how lucky I was to have a valuable family support network, but there were also friends I wasn't as close to before Teddy was sick who suddenly stepped up in a really meaningful way. It would have been easy to keep those friends at arm's length to retain more privacy: however, the value and help they brought was incredible. If you keep people at a distance they will stay at a distance. Since your heart has already been broken with this terrible diagnosis, what do you have to lose by letting people who say they want to help, help?

Before my boys were born, I was given an incredible piece of advice from a night nanny I knew. She told me to tell our visitors that they could come and visit the children but that we had only one request. Please don't feel the need to bring us presents; please bring us a meal we can reheat easily. As new parents of twins, this gave us the energy we needed to function through sleep deprivation.

When I was in hospital with Teddy before the hospital agreed to cook to my recipes and people asked how they could help, I asked for a meal for Ted and me. Yes, it felt awkward and to start with I felt like we were being a burden, but they wanted to help, and I wanted to feed Teddy properly and not ultra-processed beige garbage. You just have to feel comfortable enough with the person cooking the meals to explain the basic rules, because you can't risk the patient or anyone else getting sick – they have a compromised immune system. My long-term goal through this book is, I hope, to be able to donate pre-made super healthy but delicious meals to oncology units and their families so this stress can be removed from their overloaded pile.

The natural next question a person cooking for you to ask will be what they can bring. I used to give them one of my super easy inexpensive recipes and I think people were grateful to have the pressure of having to decide what to cook removed. But by the same token when Kurt's eighty-three-year-old grandmother spontaneously arrived to meet me in the hospital car park with her delicious homemade fish pie, that was also well received, and we were grateful.

Nor will I ever forget the day we were all home together and our friend Sylvester and his wife Claudia knocked at the door, not to come in but they had a bag of delicious goodies from Gail's bakery with a sourdough loaf and other extras. They handed Kurt the bag at the doorstep and left. I was still in my dressing gown at midday trying to manage all the madness of oncology life and I turned away from the door and sobbed. The kindness was overwhelming, and we were so touched.

You not only need to teach people how to help you in these ways, but also how to talk to you, specifically doctors. This was crucial to my anxiety levels in the early days of diagnosis and treatment. I told them… It's *when* not *if*.

None of us has a crystal ball. If we did, the lottery wouldn't exist. And I totally get why oncology teams have to be super careful what they say to their patients and their families, but the words we use can have a profound impact. I understand that there's also the insurance element and the risk of being sued, but I think sometimes we have to sit in the seat of the families going through this devastating process and hear through their ears how the words might land. Maybe it was due to the way Teddy was diagnosed but I had a distinct distrust and fear that the team knew something about Teddy's prognosis they weren't sharing. As a result, I was pretty bullish, back to fight or flight. I was here for the duration and ready to fight with every ounce of my being.

In the first few days of being admitted to our primary care oncology hospital, our lead haematology consultant and at least two other senior doctors within her team came in to see us. Something came up when we asked about the treatment plan and the first round of chemo. The response was ambivalent: "Well, *if* this works, xyz comes next."

I remember the next bit clearly because I was enraged at the way I felt they were being so cold and clinical about my son, a young child. In my usual bullish way I responded, "Can I just stop you there? When you talk about my son in my company, do not say *if*, say *when*. The words you say will not change the outcome and no one knows what's around the corner, but you will change the way you make me feel." My child was not a statistic, and he was not just a patient number.

Even before we knew Teddy would have to have a transplant, Kurt and I made a conscious decision that he would handle the medical 'stuff' and I would look after the wellness and the nutrition, although of course there was a cross over as both of us would have to converse with doctors on a daily basis. I knew I didn't want a single person to give me statistics or information of that nature. I was scared to hear it. Unless the answer was ninety-nine percent favourable, which it wasn't going to be, having researched AML leukaemia when he was first diagnosed, I didn't want to hear it.

Kurt protected me from certain information. Approximately sixteen months post-transplant, when I had a clear out, I found hospital paperwork and statistics relating to the genetic makeup of his cancer saying that Teddy's prognosis was only thirteen percent. If I had known that number, I don't know if I could have remained focused on the nutrition and wellness goals I was leading with. Boy, did Teddy prove those statistics wrong.

Where possible, I recommend your immediate family share out the areas of responsibility based on everyone's strengths and vulnerabilities. For example, Kurt took Teddy when he had his first general anaesthetic because I couldn't handle the idea of watching our child be put to sleep. Kurt now really struggles to set foot in the hospital, so I do most of the post-transplant medical appointments. We can do the most good, for the aspects that are in our control, when we lean into our strengths.

There are also some wonderful charities out there that provide practical and financial support to families. When we were first admitted to our oncology hospital, a lovely lady came to visit and asked if we had enough money to pay our bills. When a child receives a cancer diagnosis one parent often has to stop working. However, due to my chosen career I was able to work from anywhere and Kurt and I made it work.

I'm sure some people would judge me for working from Teddy's hospital bedside, but doing so kept my head straight and allowed me to keep bringing in money to fund the additional supportive treatments and hire naturopathic doctors. I was lucky that I had an understanding client. I totally recognise the huge privilege that continuing to earn money afforded me to provide more for my child. Without that, this book wouldn't exist because everything in it I learned from experts on this journey.

The charity who looked after us in the UK was Young Lives vs Cancer. They helped us with things like getting a blue badge for Teddy so we could park more conveniently and shared with us options of support by way of benefits from the state. Luckily, we didn't need those, but the charity was really generous with their knowledge and helped us understand what was available to us as a family battling cancer.

Sometimes, little things can help you manage your stress levels. There were some small but practical things that I did for myself both in hospital and at home. Whilst I spent almost every waking moment watching, reading and learning about different things I could do to help Teddy, there were of course times when my brain was full, and I needed to unwind and just forget about cancer. Not that you can ever really forget with the beeping machines all around you, but sometimes we need to turn down the outside noise.

I am, for my sins, a lover of trashy reality TV. *Real Housewives* is my vice of choice. It's an easy watch. When the twins would nap during the pandemic as babies, I loved lying on the sofa with my first actual hot drink of the day and soaking in all the drama. But during Teddy's treatment I found that I couldn't watch it. The worry and drama in our day-to-day lives meant that my anxiety was heightened even more by all the drama on screen. So, I stuck to comedy. After all, they do say laughter is the best medicine.

I think being cautious of what you expose yourself to across all media is important. Online newspapers and social media want to keep you consuming their content for longer as this allows them to sell more ad space. They do this by using algorithms based on your preference. If you read an article about a poor young mother with terminal cancer, misdiagnosed after months of health complaints and leaving behind two young children, that's what you will see more of: cancer stories.

One of the reasons, prior to plucking up the courage to write this book, I decided to keep Teddy's social media accounts going was, so people had a place for hope. To see regular updates about a child who was doing well despite the horrific diagnosis bestowed upon him. It is why I continued (and continue) to post even after ringing the end of treatment bell.

Lying in the hospital bed in the dark just after Teddy was diagnosed, I searched on social media for my inspiration and my hope, for a child like mine that had beaten AML leukaemia and was living a happy and fulfilled normal life. I found nothing. Lots of my oncology community, including people I have made friends with, have also decided to walk away after completing treatment. I totally respect that, and this was what Kurt wanted. I just feel I owe it to the mums coming up behind me to stay.

At this point, I think it is really important to touch on anxiety and panic attacks, which can happen during this journey. I only had two panic attacks. Both times, it took place when we were in total isolation for prolonged periods of time and wasn't necessarily a reflection of Ted's health. When the mind is not busy, it can wander off into many worrying thoughts, and worry makes your brain go back to where it feels safe. Ironically, as my hypnotherapist Paul taught me, when you are in the oncology journey this means going back to the worst-case scenario. Christ knows why the brain feels safe there. You can read about the things Paul and hypnotherapy have taught me shortly.

You can do practical things to temper the feelings of anxiety. Sleep plays a huge role in my anxiety level and always has done. I also have to be pretty measured with my alcohol consumption because a mild hangover can make me catastrophise pretty much everything. Sleep is broken while you are in hospital and never of great quality. Some days, when the road isn't smooth or you are waiting on results, the anxiety can bubble and feel quite debilitating. That's ok. Your team are there to support you and they understand if you have an emotional meltdown and a cry. It makes us human. When I was waiting for Teddy's results to come back from his bone marrow biopsies to check he was still cancer free, many times the smallest thing would make me spiral. I created a little one-minute hack that you can even do hiding in the bathroom if you have little ones running around wanting your attention, like I did.

I would grab my phone, open the notes app and for a minute I would do what's called free writing. You just write and write and write and don't allow yourself to stop. I did it in bullet points. These are some actual personal examples that I have never really shared before. I started every line off with *Teddy is...*

Teddy is healthy.
Teddy's immune system is strong.
Teddy is supported by supplements.
Teddy is not like the stories we hear.
Teddy's job in this life is to teach people what is possible.
Teddy went into remission in round one with zero blasts.
Teddy is a normal child going through normal things.
Teddy's doctors are thrilled with his progress.
Teddy is a survivor.

This is an exact extract from my writing on 17th March 2023 when I was clearly not having a great day. I think we can thank the British weather and post-pandemic flare up of viruses for that.

I also have for you a fifteen-minute hack to use in periods of anxiety. Get some earphones and your smartphone. Go to YouTube and search for a fifteen-minute meditation for energy. I appreciate this means finding a gap, but it's really worth it if you can. While I appreciate meditation might feel alien to some people, it is said to be really good at reducing muscle tension, promoting inner wellbeing, increasing resilience to stressful situations and reducing anxiety. I sometimes did this if I woke up before Teddy and noticed that if I could fit this in during the morning it set me up well for the day. I recommend you give it a try. It can be free, but you can get paid apps if you enjoy it. Practise daily if you can for twenty-one days to create a positive habit that might help you navigate this hideous journey a little better.

Many people use counselling services when they or a loved one are going through treatments, or perhaps after it. For me, counselling during Ted's treatment was just another thing added to my plate that I didn't need. It was another thing to coordinate. Talking therapy didn't do much for me, to be honest. I'm sure it helps many, but my brain had shut down any ability to accept that my child was gravely unwell and could have died. I struggled internally just now to just write that word *died*. My brain can't accept it.

At the time, it was almost in denial, like we were just managing a common cold, and everything was going to be ok. No amount of talking to a therapist was going to change that.

However, talking therapy did help me manage my stress in the lead up to a year post-transplant. That period was quite a precarious time, and therapy enabled me to accept that my feelings were those of a lioness there to protect her cub. The lioness inside of me felt anxiety because she never wanted to be caught off guard again. She always wanted to be one step ahead.

Accepting the lioness and her purpose helped a little, but the real progress for me was when I was introduced to hypnotherapy by my lovely oncology mum friend, Vicky. She introduced us to Paul, who has been a vital part of my recovery and Kurt's recovery, helped us understand our brains and helped get us out of fight or flight mode.

You might find hypnotherapy similarly helpful. Perhaps you will prefer more traditional counselling services. This is likely to be a very personal choice.

CHAPTER 7

SLEEP

"Sleep is not for the weak;
it's for the wise."

- Unknown

Sleep is crucial to our survival in so many ways, for both our physical and our mental health. However, I think it goes without saying that right now good quality sleep is somewhat lacking in your life. Perhaps your brain just won't let you rest when your head hits your pillow due to a recent diagnosis for you or someone you love, despite your physical and mental exhaustion. Maybe you are currently in a hospital environment where your sleep is regularly disturbed. In this chapter you'll find my helpful hints and tips to get the best possible *quality* of sleep, even if the amount is nowhere near what it ought to be.

The importance of a good night's sleep is a tale as old as time, whether we're talking about a new mum and her growing baby, a school age child, or someone under incredible stress and pressure. I am a terrible sleeper in as much as I can survive and function on very little sleep and I wake at a pin drop. Even when the twins were born and they said to sleep when the babies slept, I just couldn't. If it's 'daytime hours' my body won't let me nap. This is probably partly down to how I was brought up: going for a nap in the daytime was perceived as being a bit lazy whilst the rest of the household was on the go doing chores. This is ironic really, given that my German mother's answer to every minor ailment was to go to bed early with a cup of chamomile tea. You might feel the way I did when Teddy got sick – that you can't prioritise sleep because an hour slept is an hour not spent researching the things you have not yet found that contain something to steer you fast in the surefire direction of cure.

I didn't have this book to give me ideas and plans and hope. This is why I have written this book for you. I don't want you to miss out on sleep as much as I did or felt I had to. I wish I had known the direct impact sleep has on stress and how it can help you empty some of your stress bucket. This is another incredible thing that Paul, my hypnotherapist, has taught me about the brain.

Paul explained to me that your brain is like a video recorder during the day. You are recording everything but not processing it yet, just holding it in storage for later. When you go into an REM (Rapid Eye Movement) sleep state or a meditation or hypnotic state of trance, the brain starts processing and organising that information.

REM is one of your body's five stages of sleep.

During REM, your brain activity increases, and you can have vivid dreams. It plays a crucial role in your emotional regulation, cognitive function and memory. Alcohol can have a negative effect on the REM cycle. Although you might fall asleep faster, it disrupts the sleep cycle and affects the amount of REM sleep you get. You can even get a rebound effect whereby your stress levels plus alcohol have a negative impact on your REM cycle, causing more nightmares.

With a good bedtime routine and a good number of sleeping hours, an adult can normally achieve about 20-25 percent of total sleep time in REM. The first cycle is usually the shortest and starts approximately ninety minutes after you fall asleep. Then you have multiple REM cycles through the night, the last one being the longest. This explains why being disrupted at four am by a small child or a nurse in hospital can make you feel truly hideous the next day.

Another way Paul explained the technical elements of REM to me was to think about your bedroom. During the day you mess up your bedroom with new stuff coming in such as things you have bought on a shopping spree. You pile all these in the centre of your room. In the first stages of sleep that night, you go into your cupboards and shelves and organise what's already there to make space for the new stuff. This is called NREM. In the latter stages of sleep you take the new stuff you have bought and organise it on the shelves so you can start the next day with a clean bedroom. This is why Paul says that when people aren't able or don't choose to get enough sleep, their brains are very cluttered, and they aren't able to organise things. They risk thinking about things in a fuzzy way. When the brain is overwhelmed because it's not organising things, it stays in a state of flight or fight because it doesn't have the capacity to manage it all.

So, a parent who is trying to care for their child with cancer and who isn't getting enough sleep, which is difficult to juggle, will struggle with decision making.

Of course, getting enough sleep is difficult when you are worried and stressed and on an oncology journey either for yourself or someone else, but you do have to try. For everyone's sake.

Create an environment that supports good sleep to set yourself up for success. I understand it might feel like just another thing to add to your to-do list but even doing some of these things creates the potential to change the way you feel the next day and give you some inner strength.

Train your brain that it's almost time to go to sleep by having a good routine before you go to bed. Your brain will learn over time what is expected. When we were in hospital, after I finished my research for the night, I would put my pyjamas on and spend five minutes taking some vitamins and putting moisturiser on. I had never had a skincare routine before, and I don't particularly have one now, but it became a robotic process that I did night after night.

It is recommended that you don't use screens for an hour before bed because of the impact the blue lights can have on your brain, disrupting your winding down before bed. Personally, I wasn't willing to give this up. I usually sat in the dark whilst Teddy was already sleeping. I couldn't leave our room and go for a walk or sit and read a book with a light on. You can get blue light blockers either in the form of a sticker for your phone or glasses. I am considering glasses for myself to see if they make a difference.

One of the best products I took to hospital was a simple 3D eye mask that covers your eyes and the area around them. I already had a pair at home which we bought around the time we were doing a loft extension and didn't have any blinds. I won't be without them now and I use them when Kurt chooses to stay up later than me, doom scrolling or watching TV in bed. I also use them during my hypnotherapy sessions with Paul as I struggle to get into a rested state without being in pure darkness. I would recommend you try them. They are inexpensive and I would gift these to anyone spending a night in hospital to help them get a better night's sleep.

Another way to support a good night's sleep that can be free is to use sound frequencies or sleep meditations either through your favourite streaming site or YouTube. Personally, I didn't use headphones as I worried, I wouldn't hear Ted if he needed me. Playing it out loud in our private hospital room meant he might have benefitted from them as well.

Search for long-form videos of eight hours or more, using search terms like 'sleep meditation for healing' or 'sound waves between 100hz and 300hz'. There is some research into sonodynamic (sound based) therapies, investigating sound waves and their impact on cancerous cells, encouraging them to commit cell suicide at that frequency. It is very new research and there are not many of studies on it yet. The work that has been done so far is mainly on cells in a lab (in vitro) and with animals.

Let's be honest: I can't see them ever adding that to an oncology treatment plan and it's certainly not a conventional treatment replacement. But that's not why I did it; I only found out about this research much later. I used sleep meditations at a stressful time in my life with great success in feeling rested the next morning. I also found it helped my children drift off to sleep better in those challenging toddler years. I just have to be careful I don't fall asleep myself as I've woken up many times with a sore back having drifted off whilst putting the boys down.

My attitude is that if it can't harm but could benefit, especially when it comes to cancer, chuck the kitchen sink at it. Although we have focused on the mental health benefits of sleep so far in this chapter, there are huge physical benefits to a good night's sleep.

Physical benefits include improved immune function, reduced inflammation, detoxification, pain relief, and muscle recovery and growth to name just a few. When you get a good night's sleep, your body's cells recreate as new, they repair, and they improve their functional abilities. Old and damaged cells are replaced with new, healthy ones.

Research tells us that people with an irregular sleep pattern may have an increased risk of developing cancer due to the impact on the body's natural sleep and awake rhythm (the circadian rhythm). The circadian rhythm not only controls our sleep-wake windows but our hormone release processes including melatonin (which helps you sleep) and cortisol (stress hormone). It supports your mood, brain function and immune system, which is why many recommend that shift workers prioritise sleep, diet and stress management.

I did other things in hospital to improve the quality of our sleep and to reduce my and Teddy's stress levels, some of which I appreciate might raise eyebrows. In the previous chapter, I touched upon the importance of reducing stress to allow the body's healing process to be uninhibited. I banned anyone from taking Teddy's blood pressure between ten pm and six am. This was agreed so long as Teddy had a healthy blood pressure at the last check.

You may already know that nurses are required to do regular observations, shortened to obs, on their patients in terms of heart rates, oxygen levels, blood pressure and temperature. Early into our diagnosis, we had several days of Teddy having had literally no sleep due to being constantly woken up due to the blood pressure machine they attach to the arm or leg. Someone I knew well had been taken to hospital in the Middle East following a seizure and had mentioned how the doctors wanted them to rest, and so they had been allowed to sleep and not be disturbed by having the BP reading taken at night. I asked a senior doctor what would happen if Teddy didn't have his blood pressure reading taken at night.

The doctor replied that whilst it was not ideal, as long as they could monitor heart rate and those other obs, the risks were relatively small. And that was it, Teddy never had another BP reading again at night. I refused them all in every setting. We kept him on a monitor that checked his heart rate and oxygen levels, attached to his toe via a sticking plaster that hospitals carry for young children. The temperature check using the ear thermometer was easily carried out without waking him. Of course, it didn't mean he was never disturbed of a night but that was often due to a mishap or waking of his own accord or a noise that threw off his sleep.

I understand why hospitals insist on doing obs through the night for insurance reasons. However, I was lucky our doctors were also reasonable and pragmatic people who wanted the best for Teddy, and they knew the importance of good sleep, not only for his physical body but for his temperament and compliance with treatment the next day. We were working together as a team, and they didn't feel they had grounds to refuse the request given how well he was doing. That partnership and willingness to compromise meant that had they ever pushed to take the BP in the night, I wouldn't have refused.

I also made sure I knew what to expect from our schedule throughout the day so I could protect his daytime naps. I adjusted his positioning to make sure his connecting wires were reachable, and it didn't affect what the nurses needed to do. However, I did send nurses away who attempted obs off-schedule and put a polite – perhaps slightly passive-aggressive sign – on our door to advise them that a small child was napping and to be quiet upon entry.

Teddy also had Reiki every other week with our Reiki master, Reeya Avani, which contributed hugely to the quality of his sleep. I would normally place Reiki in the complementary therapies chapter, but the impact on his sleep was so profound that it would be wrong to exclude it from this chapter.

When we were being supported by Reeya through treatment, there was a big press debacle about a UK-based cancer hospital advertising for a Reiki practitioner to support oncology patients on a salary from taxpayer money. Since it is a complementary therapy and the National Health Service is struggling, the media created a storm claiming that people weren't happy about it and felt it didn't have enough value.

Reeya was asked onto live TV not once but twice in the space of a week and I was asked to share our experiences on air as a patient. Teddy was taking a medication known to cause insomnia, but whenever that child had a Reiki session he would sleep for hours and hours. If I could have afforded it, Teddy would have had Reiki every day. Say what you will about a placebo effect, an eighteen-month-old doesn't understand and cannot be manipulated into a placebo.

The practice of Reiki is all to do with energy, emotion and spirituality, and started in Japan in the early twentieth century. It is based on the principle that every living being or thing has a life force energy running through them called *chi*. Reiki practitioners work on the belief that this energy can help heal the body and the mind.

I had tried Reiki before due to personal circumstances in my old life and I was one of the lucky ones with the means to chuck the kitchen sink at cancer and hit it from every possible angle. I found Reeya, having discovered that she was one of the best in the country, and left her a ridiculous, blubbering voicemail explaining how I needed her help. She texted me to say that she was on route to her Easter holidays but felt compelled to get in touch and that she would help me where she could as soon as she was home.

Reeya is now more like family than part of our support system. Teddy is not very trusting of adults, particularly post-treatment, even of nurses he likes, but when he last saw Reeya he happily popped on her lap for a cuddle. He rarely does that with anyone. They feel very bonded, and I think that has helped the sessions he's had with her to be a success. In these instances, you have to be trusting and feel connected otherwise (in my case) you could end up with a toddler running around a room going buck wild.

Research in Reiki is limited to date but the anecdotal evidence from the research I did with other people who had Reiki and the TV programmes I took part in all seems to align between patients. Benefits included less stress and anxiety and better emotional health, being able to relax at a deeper level, pain relief (which could be due to mind over matter), clearer thinking and better quality of sleep. From my experience, Reiki is certainly a way to promote balance within the body and relax better. Countries who follow Eastern medicine use it frequently. Whilst not yet widely accepted in Western medicine, I do think it has value by way of supporting a cancer patient in terms of wellbeing, should your budget allow. If not, you can source great Reiki tracks that you could use in place of sleep meditation. They could also support a good night's sleep and therefore potentially help elements of recovery.

Outside of this, I did a couple of other things during our oncology journey and there are practices I have implemented afterwards that form part of our standard routine. The first is that I try my best last thing at night to think about all the positive things that happened that day, not necessarily to do with cancer. I might be really proud of how I managed that difficult conversation with so and so: I'm really learning how to manage my emotions better. Or I'm pleased I made the time to eat properly today; it's hard to put myself first. I try to bring to the front of my mind, before I go to sleep either with or without a sleep meditation, anything positive or any little thing that either child or my husband did.

During times when I was looking for a way to unwind, I would also start pricing up trips I wanted to take the children on in the future. The night before Teddy received his stem cell transplant, I was imagining taking the boys on a safari to celebrate Teddy's five-year post-transplant anniversary. I visualised and pictured our future down to where we would stay, what we would do, how much it would cost and the boys' faces seeing all the animals in the wild. It was not only a great distraction but felt like a manifestation or a prediction of the future – a million miles away from the present which was what my brain needed.

It is all too easy for people to say those impacted by cancer should think positively. Such advice can feel very patronising to those of us who are living it. I would say, celebrate the little wins where you can, allow yourself to daydream about events and make your mind paint a picture of them, but don't feel bad on the days when you can't get out of the funk and see the positives. Going through an oncology journey yourself or with someone you love is a roller coaster of emotions that change daily.

Staying in hospital is not a lot of fun, even without the awful itchy sheets and paper-thin blankets. I totally understand that it comes down to funding and running costs, but if you have ever had to spend a night in hospital you know that if it's not the bright lights and noises keeping you awake, it is the fact that you do not feel particularly warm and cosy. When we went in for transplant, we brought our own pillows and duvets but used hospital sheets. Our covers had to be washed daily due to transplant rules and risk of infection which was a lot of work but well worth it.

Knowing what I know now, if I had my time again, I would have also brought in the grounding sheets that I have on all our beds at home under our sheets, having learned about grounding (otherwise known as earthing). But I only learned about this practice after Ted's transplant.

The principle of grounding is that humans are electrical beings, and we need to be physically connected to the earth's electrical energy. By being physically connected to nature via direct contact, it is claimed that our bodies are able to absorb the natural electric charge that it gives off and the process helps balance out the harmful particles in our body called free radicals. Free radicals are known to cause inflammation and other health issues.

Please don't think I have gone too far on the woo-woo scale and close the book. There are already well over twenty scientific studies on earthing which have looked at the effects on inflammation and related health outcomes. It is all really positive, but more work needs to be done in this area, for sure. Scientists appear to be quite interested in how grounding has been evidenced, through diagnostic tools like scans, to lower inflammation markers and pain, promote healing and improve sleep quality.

Most people practise grounding by spending time walking barefoot in nature, whether that's walking on grass or taking a walk through the woods which is what I recently did with my children. I've added some of these studies to the further reading chapter and there is also a documentary film called *The Earthing Movie* that you might enjoy watching. You can find it free online.

Recently, there has been a big uptake in people's interest in how they can ground themselves better in their day-to-day lives whilst often being removed from nature due to work and responsibilities. We don't all have time or space to walk barefoot in nature, so companies have found ways to potentially deliver the same results at home through products such as grounding mats and grounding sheets.

Grounding sheets, which are what I use, are usually made of cotton or silver material and they are usually attached to a plug that by only connects to the earthing element of your outlet. Don't worry, you aren't at risk of electrocution. I noticed almost instantaneously that the quality of my sleep went up even when the amount I was able to get was limited. My husband also noticed a benefit. He silently supports me, but for sure thinks some of my ideas are a little bit too far out there until he tries them for himself.

I now notice immediately if my sheets plug has been accidentally turned off and I also notice it with the children. For them, the results were not immediate and took a few weeks, but they sleep better and for longer so we will continue with it. If I had my time again in hospitals, I would use grounding sheets or a grounding mat daily with Ted. The data based on tests is just too strong for me to ignore in terms of reduction of inflammation. Cancer can be associated with (although not solely) inflammation. I am not saying that using grounding sheets will impact the outcome of a diagnosis. However, because of the physical benefit of sleep that science tells us about, if grounding sheets or indeed any of the other practices help you achieve a better quality of sleep, it's always worth a try.

CHAPTER 8

COMPLEMENTARY THERAPIES

"Health is a state of complete harmony of the body, mind, and spirit."

- B.K.S. Iyengar

The foundational principles outlined in earlier chapters, such as reducing stress, ensuring quality sleep, and consuming nutrient-dense foods, serve as the groundwork for a strong immune system. This foundation is crucial for withstanding unexpected challenges such as serious side effects from conventional oncology treatments. It is also key for those trying to improve their health to prevent disease.

While some people may seek only natural or holistic treatment methods following a terminal diagnosis or before undergoing chemotherapy or radiation, I believe in integrating traditional and holistic approaches, especially for Teddy. Each option is valid for adults capable of making informed decisions, but combining both methods is often beneficial. Nature itself does not aim to harm, and you can achieve a balance with the right strategies.

Complementary therapies are so named because they are intended to be in addition to or to contribute extra beneficial features. I would never suggest anyone ever attempts to cure their cancer without traditional medicines.

In discussing the strategies, I implemented to support Teddy, I think of the body as an ecosystem with interconnected parts, aiming to maintain physical, physiological, mental and spiritual balance. Cancer is an emotionally charged subject, and my intention in sharing this information is to empower you and help you find a sense of balance amid the chaos without overwhelming.

I have learned strategies that may support the body in achieving balance, ultimately enhancing the immune system. These include methods I employed during Teddy's treatment and others I discovered afterward. Some approaches were not suitable for Teddy due to his age, but I would consider them as he gets older, should he be open to them.

If you are in treatment, it's crucial to engage with your oncology team regarding any complementary therapies you are considering. Transparent communication is vital to ensure that these therapies complement, rather than interfere with, conventional treatments. As new drugs emerge, monitoring for potential interactions is essential for your safety.

Some may be surprised by the absence of cannabis oil and the Gerson method in my recommendations. While I acknowledge the promising studies around cannabis oil and its growing acceptance in medical settings, its legality varies by location, and it is not permitted where I live. During our journey, I explored this option, even considering a trip to the U.S. to pursue it for Teddy. However, I opted against it. With over one hundred cannabinoids identified in cannabis, it is a highly complex option, and the effects can vary for each individual. If you choose this path, it's essential to work under the guidance of an oncologist who is legally allowed to prescribe it. For reliable advice, I recommend reaching out to Dr Donald Abrams, featured in the documentary "Weed the People". It centres around children going through cancer treatment who had a bleak prognosis and their journey of taking cannabis oil.

The Gerson method, introduced by Dr Max Gerson in the 1920s, advocates for a holistic approach to treatment, primarily using organic fruits, vegetables and juices. While there are some similarities with my own principles, I believe that any adoption of the Gerson therapy should be supervised by a qualified healthcare professional. Gerson's programme includes consuming thirteen juices daily and using coffee enemas for liver support, which can be beneficial for adults when properly managed at licensed centres like the one in Tijuana, Mexico, or through organisations like Hope4Cancer.

Let's delve into the complementary therapies I used and considered with Teddy, both during and post treatment. I have placed them in alphabetical order to help you use this later as a quick reference guide for further research.

FASTING

The words, "Cancer feeds on sugar," get bandied about frequently. In the 1920s, scientist Otto Warburg made an observation about cancerous cells and glucose. Depending on the cell type and its condition, it has been suggested that cancerous cells could consume up to ten times more the glucose than that of healthy cells. This characteristic is very much exploited by medical imaging including PET scans. A radioactive glucose solution is given to the patient prior to being scanned in an attempt to 'light up' cancerous cells and tumours within the body. This phenomenon has now been coined the Warburg effect.

When you think about your diet plans, I suggest you don't just look into your traditional sugars but also the volume of carbohydrates you consume, as carbs break down into sugars as part of the digestive process. Do those carbohydrates add real nutritional value or are they simply empty calories? You want to aim for wholegrains and vegetables over breads and pastas.

So how could fasting have a positive impact, either in the prevention or the treatment of cancer?

When you fast (i.e. not eating and drinking only water or herbal teas) it is reported that the body starts to look for new energy sources due to less nutrient availability. With the claim that cancerous cells rely heavily on glucose, there is the potential that cancerous cells may struggle to survive and grow during fasting periods.

In addition, the process of autophagy takes place during the fasting process. Autophagy is where cells break down and recycle damaged parts to survive. This benefits healthy cells by encouraging their repair and longevity. Cancer cells may not behave in the same way as normal cells, which in some cases could lead to cancer cell death.

Research has also indicated that fasting is helpful for your digestive system and gives your body a break to focus its energy on areas that need it most. A study published in the journal of Nutritional Science in 2019 highlighted the importance of fasting for the gut microbiome and how it can trigger positive impacts on the immune system.

How long to fast for optimal effects really does differ from person to person. However, the data I have reviewed suggests ideally fasting for seventeen hours or more if you want the key benefits when undergoing cancer treatment. Fasting for seventeen hours or more is said to help clean up cells and stimulate apoptosis. Apoptosis (see also Chapter 4) is cancerous cell suicide without negatively impacting healthy cells.

A 2016 study carried out with two thousand breast cancer patients took two groups, one of which had to fast for thirteen hours every night. They made no changes to those individuals' diets; they just had them fast. Interestingly, the group who fasted every day had sixty-four percent less recurrence of breast cancer than the control group. You would be hard pushed to find a drug that claims to achieve such results.

When Teddy was first diagnosed, I learned about the benefits of fasting from some of the communities I joined, albeit they were largely focused on adults. It made a lot of sense to me. When a young child or infant is sick, they often don't eat. Their bodies know to rest. But the rest of us see having appetite as a sign of health and are obsessed with having people eat. However, that being said, it's not easy to implement fasting with a small child. Who is going to say no to a child who wants to eat, especially one undergoing cancer treatment? I tried to work with Teddy's body and his wants, as much as possible, to create as big a fasting window as he could tolerate. Today that looks like feeding him and his brother their dinner as soon as possible when they arrive home after four pm and stretching out breakfast until as late as possible without making us late for preschool.

I know some people look to do a much longer fast during chemotherapy cycles due to claims that this helps protect healthy cells from chemo related toxicity whilst also supporting chemotherapy effectiveness. Given Teddy was under two, this wasn't really an option for us.

As with all the scientific studies and research that underpin the principles of our strategy as set out in this book, I have added more information and research papers to the further reading chapter.

If you are looking for more information on fasting, I encourage you to explore the work of Dr Mindy Pelz. She is a functional and nutritional health expert who has worked for many decades on supporting women with their health. Although focusing on women's health, her knowledge is transferable across age ranges and genders. She is the best expert I know of when it comes to fasting safely for health.

GROUNDING OR EARTHING

Grounding, also known as earthing, is a practice of connecting your body with Earth's natural energy by bringing your body into direct contact with the ground. You can do this easily by walking barefoot on grass, sand or soil or even laying down on the earth with bare skin touching the surface. Since the discovery of the potentially huge benefits of grounding as a way to naturally reduce inflammation, a number of companies have set out to create products that allow people to achieve the benefits while barely having to leave their home or their bed.

The concept is based on the idea that the Earth has a negative charge, and that connecting the body with it can help balance the body's electrical system. It is said that when a body is grounded, the electrons from the earth are absorbed and that these electrons act as antioxidants and could help remove free radicals that cause oxidative stress and inflammation in the body.

Several studies have explored the effects of grounding on inflammation and related health conditions. For instance, research has shown that grounding can lead to a reduction in your blood's thickness, a factor linked to cardiovascular health and inflammation. A study published in the Journal of Inflammation Research indicated that grounding improved blood flow and reduced markers of inflammation in the body, which may help in faster recovery from exercise and injury.

Furthermore, some studies have suggested that grounding may positively influence cortisol levels, the hormone associated with stress. Elevated cortisol can contribute to inflammation and a host of other health issues. By promoting a more relaxed state of mind and potentially lowering cortisol levels, grounding may facilitate a decrease in inflammation.

Based on the science and the research carried out to date, grounding could hold a great deal of potential for cancer patients for several reasons:

1. **Reduced inflammation** – Chronic inflammation has been widely recognised as a significant factor contributing to the development of cancer and its progression.
2. **Better wellbeing** – It has been reported that grounding has benefited people by reducing their stress and anxiety levels. We know that experiencing a cancer diagnosis is incredibly distressing for both the patient and their loved ones so anything that supports emotional wellbeing is surely a plus.
3. **Improved quality of sleep** – Several studies have focused on the impact of grounding and sleep and its potential to improve the quality of sleep. We all know sleep is crucial to giving the body rest to recover and allow medications to do their best work. This is why I have never understood the rationale for disturbing cancer patients in hospitals whilst they are sleeping.

I watched *The Earthing Movie* during my research. It is a fascinating documentary, packed full of science and an easy watch to help me grasp the principles of grounding. I highly recommend you seek it out so you can learn more than my brief introduction. The children and I still love to ground ourselves to the earth by walking barefoot in nature whenever the weather allows us to. It is very calming and with two toddlers who love to run at high speed, I don't know why I didn't consider whipping off their shoes and socks sooner and having them walk barefoot through the woods. It certainly slows them down. Where we live is very seasonal and often cold and wet, so we also use grounding sheets on our bed which I love, as does my husband.

He's used to me sharing yet another practice I want to try and for the most part he's a good sport. He's just a 'to see is to believe' type of person. When I first started talking to him about the importance of grounding, he kind of rolled his eyes and muttered a few half-supportive grunts. So, he did lift a questioning eyebrow when he climbed into bed one evening to find his favourite Egyptian cotton sheets had been replaced with a tartan-like beige sheet with a button in the corner and a strange looking wire hanging down from it that connected to the plug in the wall. That is, until he started having the best possible sleep even when the number of hours we slept was shortened.

Our boys were three at the time and Teddy was going through a phase of wanting to come into our bed at night. Hence, I bought the grounding sheets for all of us to see if we could benefit with better and more restful sleep as per the claims. I certainly would have taken them to hospital whilst we were inpatient had I known. Sleep matters. Whilst I don't have access to tests to evidence the before and after of my family's inflammation levels, I do know that sleep matters for your health… your mental health and your stress levels, but also your physical health and giving your body time to shut down and repair itself. And if it is true that grounding can address the killer silent inflammation as well, that sounds like a winning practice with no required cost or risk.

HOMEOPATHY

Homeopathy operates on the principle of 'like cures like', similar to how traditional medicine prescribes stimulants for individuals with ADHD to help them focus. It involves administering highly diluted substances that, in larger amounts, would produce symptoms similar to those being treated.

The practice originated in the eighteenth century with Dr Samuel Hahnemann, who sought gentler and more effective treatments. Homeopathy has gained significant popularity in countries like India, France and Germany, and it was even utilised by the NHS until 2017, when it was removed due to claims of insufficient evidence backing its efficacy. However, many people still turn to homeopathy for children's ailments and chronic conditions across Europe, and homeopathic medicines must comply with safety and quality standards under the Medicines Act in the UK.

Advocacy for homeopathy can be traced back to the royal family since the time of George VI. In 1993, as Prince of Wales, King Charles established The Prince's Foundation for Integrated Health to promote complementary and alternative medicine, including lobbying for its integration into the NHS. In 2023, his appointment of Dr Mike Dixon, a pro-homeopathy doctor, as head of the royal medical household further highlights this support, although Dixon emphasises that while homeopathy does not cure cancer, complementary therapies can aid conventional treatments safely and effectively.

On a related topic, in my previous canine nutrition business, we sold nosodes as vaccine alternatives, providing diluted substances derived from the disease's vaccines aim to protect against without incorporating harmful chemicals. My dogs had their puppy vaccines, and I then opted for titre tests to evaluate their immunity instead of re-vaccinating. I believe in the concept of immune memory. After Teddy's bone marrow transplant, the medical team recommended redoing all childhood vaccinations. I insisted on antibody tests before proceeding. When the results showed that he retained immunity to certain diseases, I chose not to re-vaccinate him immediately due to concerns regarding heavy metal exposure and its potential impact on his development.

Homeopathy has played a significant role in my life, particularly during my son's treatment. For example, arnica is commonly known as a homeopathic remedy for bruises and inflammation. To navigate life after treatment, we recently enlisted a skilled homeopath named Dawn, who specialises in support for oncology patients. I wish we had consulted her sooner.

Dawn's background as an oncology nurse at a leading children's hospital enhances my trust in her expertise. Recently, when Teddy caught yet another cold, she provided homeopathic remedies to alleviate his symptoms without resorting to antibiotics. During a recent hospital check-up, Teddy's blood results were the best they have ever been, with healthy white blood cell counts. In the past these would have been high in response to the cold, which typically would have prompted discussions to start the use of antibiotics.

One of my only regrets during this journey is allowing George to return to nursery during winter, which inadvertently exposed Teddy to winter germs and numerous fevers. Whilst our hospital encouraged it, I really regret not thinking it through more. This resulted in a reliance on antibiotics, which I believe have negatively impacted his gut health and immune system. Fortunately, with guidance from Dawn and Dr Kate, and through our commitment to a varied and diverse diet, we are working to strengthen Teddy's immune system.

Teddy has generally coped well with common illnesses, so much so that a shared care consultant once discharged him from the ward at six months post-transplant, within forty eight hours, due to his remarkable wellbeing, despite having the flu. I can't help but wonder if we could have avoided numerous hospital admissions and antibiotic treatments with earlier input from Dawn. Now, my medicine cabinet is stocked with homoeopathic remedies, and I will continue to use them as a primary line of defence for common ailments.

Looking back, my experience highlights the potential benefits of homeopathy as a complementary therapy. It offers a gentle, effective approach that can coexist with conventional treatments, supporting overall health and wellbeing.

HYPERBARIC OXYGEN THERAPY (HBOT)

Hyperbaric Oxygen Therapy (HBOT) is a medical treatment that involves breathing one hundred percent oxygen in a specially designed chamber at pressures typically two or three times higher than normal air pressure. This environment allows increased oxygen concentration to go into the bloodstream and tissues with the aim of enhancing the body's own healing processes. There are many promising studies and research coming out on the use of HBOT to support stroke victims, individuals with autism and cancer patients.

Every living being on the plant and every living cell needs oxygen to stay alive and thrive. In patients with cancer, maintaining optimal oxygen levels is critical. This is probably why you are encouraged to exercise when you feel well and able to do so, because when we exercise, we increase circulation of oxygen levels in the body. Cancer cells tend to thrive in low-oxygen environments while being less capable of surviving in oxygen-rich conditions.

HBOT is said to have the potential to disrupt tumour growth by boosting the oxygen going to tissues, which could help slow cancer growth and improve treatment results.

Some of the key benefits I found in my research that may benefit cancer patients included:

1. **Faster wound healing:** One of the main uses of HBOT is to speed up how wounds heal. Cancer treatments can create challenging side effects, like surgical cuts or damage from radiation. Getting more oxygen helps the body create new blood vessels and repair tissue, which is super important for getting patients back on their feet.
2. **Help with radiation damage:** Many treatment plans for oncology patients include radiation therapy, which can damage healthy tissues around the area by way of a side effect. HBOT has been shown to help those tissues bounce back from the damage and ease symptoms from radiation.

3. **Reduced inflammation:** Chronic inflammation can be a real struggle for cancer patients and make recovery tougher. HBOT can help reduce inflammation in different parts of the body, which can support healing after intense cancer treatments.
4. **Boosted stem cell production:** Exciting studies suggest that HBOT might kickstart the production of stem cells in the body. These cells are crucial for fixing and regenerating tissues, which is especially important for cancer patients trying to recover from treatment damage quickly.
5. **Strengthened immune system:** HBOT can give a boost to the immune system by helping white blood cells do their job more efficiently. This is really important for oncology patients, who often have a higher risk of infections and therefore need additional support during treatment.
6. **Brain benefits:** For patients facing brain tumours, or brain fog or cognitive issues from treatment, HBOT might help improve brain function. Getting more oxygen to the brain can help with recovery and enhance mental abilities, which is key for maintaining a good quality of life.

There is a fine balance regarding whom Hyperbaric Oxygen Therapy is suitable and not suitable for during active treatment. For some it can increase chemotherapy toxicity levels so you must discuss with your medical team. HBOT is typically not recommended during active treatment phases for some patients, but it is often viewed more favourably as a therapeutic approach following the completion of intensive treatments.

That said, I think there are many benefits after the end of treatment which is the strategy I will now look to adopt with Teddy, hoping he's now of an age where he's happy to sit in a chamber for longer periods of time whilst having screen time.

RED LIGHT THERAPY

Out of all the alternative and supportive treatments in this chapter, Near Infrared Light Therapy (NIR) is one of the few I have never personally heard of being used as an alternative therapy. It has always been used more as a supportive tool for the body alongside conventional or non-conventional treatment in terms of reducing inflammation, promoting healing, potentially reducing pain levels and improving skin health. It is currently going through a phase of being a go-to product in the beauty industry, although I'm not entirely convinced of the quality of the near infrared light face masks, I see all over my social media or that they have much of a therapeutic effect, but that's an opinion purely based on the price of the products being offered.

True near infrared light therapy is a non-invasive treatment that uses specific wavelengths of light (usually 700-1200 nanometres) using either a handheld device, a large panel or a sauna. We used a device with a cut-off timer after twelve minutes. It is said that light penetrates the skin to stimulate activity in the cells and is absorbed by the mitochondria. The device is usually used at least six inches away from a clean and naked skin. It doesn't make the skin get hot so there is no risk of sunburn. Our device was cool when I tested it on myself, but from what I understand a powerful device feels similar to when the sun's rays hit your skin on a warm but not hot day. So... just a bit cosy.

If you choose to rabbit hole into the topics in this book, I have no doubt that the term *mitochondria* will come up often. Your liver, brain and muscles rely heavily on the mitochondria for their vital functions. The mitochondria are the powerhouses found within most cells in your body. They could be thought of as tiny factories within the cells that perform several very important jobs. Not only do they take food and turn it into energy so we can function, but they also control metabolism and, most crucially from an oncology perspective, they control cell death, a process called apoptosis whereby cells basically commit suicide. This is how the body gets rid of old and damaged cells when they are no longer required. When cancer occurs, this doesn't happen as the healthy cells are unable to kill off the bad ones. (See also Chapter 4: Supplements)

The NIR light waves being consumed by the mitochondria enhances levels of ATP (Adenosine Triphosphate) in the body, which is critical for cellular repair processes and giving the cells in your body energy. Think of ATP like the fuel in your car. It allows your cells to do their basic functions or even something more strenuous like going for a run. On this basis, I can see why this could be helpful to oncology patients during treatment: whilst not affecting treatment or medication it could potentially support them when they are struggling to eat enough and are bed bound. This is before considering the claimed anti-inflammatory benefits. That being said, it's certainly not a substitute for nutrition but could be a great additional tool in your arsenal.

I was first introduced to Near Infrared Light Therapy via a lovely transplant mum called Megan from Canada who found me via social media and wanted nutrition and supplement advice. She had a NIR device for her son and he was doing great also. I now use it with both boys after bath times three to five times per week. I would most certainly have taken my small handheld device into the hospital and used it with Teddy had I known about it at that time. If your budget allows it's great to have and I'm glad to have one, but I wouldn't honestly prioritise this tool over nutrition and supplements had I been in that position. But if it's good enough for an athlete to recover from what they put their bodies through, it's good enough in the long term for Ted.

REIKI

Teddy started Reiki and crystal healing therapy soon after he was diagnosed. He had sessions once a fortnight well into his time post-treatment. It is one of my favourites both for cancer patients and their carers.

Reiki originated in Japan in the early twentieth century and is a practice centred around energy healing. Practitioners or Reiki Masters channel universal energy to work with the body's natural energy systems and can help the flow of energy to promote balance and healing.

Reiki helps release suppressed emotions, improves self-awareness and helps people move through grief.

There are two main types of Reiki practice. One is carried out in person in a clinic, but some experts are also able to carry out Reiki remotely by sending distance healing, which is something we have done for both Teddy and George.

There are seven chakras within the body that play a key role in Reiki and energy healing. Chakras are energy centres or points that play a role in your physical, mental and emotional wellbeing and help keep you balanced. They are like muscles and regularly practising Reiki is said to strengthen a person's energy field and create harmony. When these chakras are open and balanced, it's thought that you feel healthier and more in tune with yourself. If they get blocked or out of balance, you might experience physical or emotional issues. Reiki supports the flow of energy and is said to be an intelligent therapy as it knows where to go in order to unblock or heal.

One of the benefits of Reiki is that there are no reported negative side effects which is why it holds great potential for cancer patients. Some UK hospitals even employ Reiki practitioners to offer it as a complementary therapy to its patients.

There has been research and a number of studies into the benefits of Reiki to those facing both chronic and acute health conditions. I have detailed these resources in the further reading chapter, but here is a quick summary of how Reiki can support cancer patients.

1. **Pain relief:** Reiki may help ease pain, which is great for cancer patients dealing with the effects of surgery, chemo or radiation. It promotes relaxation that can lower how much pain you feel.
2. **Less anxiety and stress**: Facing cancer can greatly increase anxiety and stress. Reiki sessions are calming and can help reduce those feelings, bringing a sense of peace that's important for mental health.
3. **Better emotional wellbeing**: Reiki boosts emotional strength, helping patients cope with the tough mental challenges of cancer treatment. It promotes relaxation and balance, making it easier to handle feelings during treatment.
4. **Improved sleep:** Many cancer patients struggle with sleep issues because of pain and anxiety. Reiki has been linked to better sleep quality, which is key for recovery.

Teddy experienced huge benefits from Reiki. As a family we really noticed the difference between the days he had Reiki treatment and days he did not. Due to the medications that were part of his treatment plan, he struggled to get to sleep and stay asleep. When he had Reiki, he always slept through, and we could see the difference in his energy levels the next day.

Whilst I understand that some people might find it challenging to buy into the benefits of Reiki as they are not visible and write it off as nothing more than a placebo effect, Teddy was only eighteen months old when he started having Reiki. He couldn't understand any of the concepts for a placebo effect to be plausible. But the benefits of Reiki and use of crystals were very clear to see.

I remember being very concerned, even panicked, about Teddy's high blood pressure in the early days of treatment. He was hooked up to a monitor and the next step was going to be to start medication to force his blood pressure down. Reeya had kindly dropped a number of crystals to us at the hospital some weeks before, and when I called her and explained my worries, she recommended I put a crystal called bloodstone on his thymus (a gland on the top part of the chest between the lungs) and within an hour his blood pressure had dropped to a normal level.

Crystals, used alongside Reiki, are said to elevate the energy levels and make the sessions more powerful.

Crystal healing is a holistic practice that uses the unique properties of crystals and gemstones to promote physical, emotional and spiritual wellbeing. Each crystal is believed to have its own vibrational frequency, and the idea is that they can interact with your body's energy to help rebalance and align you. When placed on or near the body, crystals are thought to vibrate at specific frequencies, potentially helping to release negative energy, reduce stress, and support healing processes by boosting the flow of positive energy that aligns with our own body's natural energy.

We have quite the crystal collection today by adding to it slowly over time and we have adopted the practice of Reiki for the long term. In the chapter about sleep, I suggested using Reiki soundtracks whilst sleeping to support good quality sleep and wellbeing as an alternative approach if your budget doesn't allow you to work with a Reiki Master or practitioner. I highly recommend Reiki both for those on an oncology journey and those who have been through a challenging time in the past. Our emotional wellbeing plays such a vital role in our physical wellbeing that it is unwise to discount troubles as things we have to struggle through. Reiki could support you through this, your hardest time.

CHAPTER 9

QUESTION EVERYTHING

"Question everything but do it respectfully: Your right for choice."

- Sarah Cripps

You are entitled to advocate for yourself, your child or a family member.

I wrote this chapter to help you feel empowered and give you the confidence to ask the questions you feel uneasy about, and not just when a doctor gives you permission to do so. You don't need to go into every medical scenario with blind faith because someone is wearing a white coat. Nor does every interaction with a medical professional need to be combative with you looking to trip them up.

There needs to be trust but you also need to be in a position to make informed decisions. There are lots of risks to navigate constantly and try to mitigate. If you ask questions, you are then able to offer more information to your medical team so that they can make the right decisions for you or your loved one. It is impossible for your doctor to know every tiny detail about their patients and their medical history. Sometimes our interventions can stop a disaster from occurring.

In this chapter you can read about a couple of occasions when we had incidents that could have been real disasters and what I learned from them. There are also things I would never have thought to ask about (or felt too afraid to ask about medications) but the parents of other patients encouraged me. I want to pass the torch on to you. There were times I really could have been a little softer in my communication – I concede that – although I was always respectful. There is a fine line between being assertive and being rude. However, I would stress that sometimes you will have to be stubborn to the point of refusing treatment unless someone gives you the time to explain the what's and whys. It is ok to be that person. If you want to be that person but feel afraid, that's ok too. Make friends with your nurses where you can first. They can help you become as informed as possible. If, however, you are genuinely in a scary situation and you don't feel heard, I will share with you the triggers you can pull – probably what you would classify as the nuclear options.

When you first get diagnosed with leukaemia, they take a sample of the cancerous cells and send them off for genetic testing to determine the risk levels and thereby what your treatment path should be. When Teddy was first diagnosed, he was deemed standard risk, which would mean six straight rounds of chemotherapy. However, there was testing that came back later and I was told that Teddy would need a bone marrow transplant, by a junior doctor in quite hideous circumstances who was extremely clumsy in his approach.

But that's a story that doesn't need telling in detail, not because it was so bad but because it was such a small part of our journey. Whilst it was bad at the time, I'm over it.

The genetics that came back for Teddy placed him as high risk: a gene called p13. One of the worst, according to the report that categorised all the genes. I think it was called the FISH study, but I can't bear to check. That's a box I don't need to open again.

From a study of thousands (and I mean many thousands) of people, only twenty-eight had the p13 leukaemia gene. I remember that figure as Kurt wouldn't let me forget it. Kurt had no real confidence in the quality of the data, and he wasn't willing to sign a consent form until someone made him really believe this was the right thing for Teddy. On the other hand, I had always seen a transplant as a likely path to cure as my cousin Michael was always due to have a transplant to save his life. He passed away from the more common leukaemia (acute lymphoblastic leukaemia) when I was twelve.

> "So how many of these have you done before?" Kurt asked.
>
> I could feel myself cringing and squirming in my seat. I wanted to hide my face in my hands. I'd been with this man since 2012, and I knew exactly where this was going, and it was about to get incredibly uncomfortable.
>
> "A few, maybe ten." The haematologist, a very experienced and incredibly strong female in her late fifties, was squirming a little. She knew this wasn't going to be your bog-standard pre-transplant

> conversation; Kurt was going to hold her feet to the fire and be damn sure that any decision we made was the right one for our child.
>
> "So, what you are basically telling me is I am better off going down to Ladbrokes…"
>
> Kurt, no you did *not* just say that! In my head, I was screaming, "This is *cancer* not a bloody Saturday three pm kick off and an accumulator."

To be fair to Kurt, he had good reason to be concerned. He understands data as he works with it every day and had even asked some of his team to do some data analysis prior to the meeting. The hospital's data on Ted's leukaemia genetics, he said, was completely flawed and with a ten percent chance of losing Ted as part of the transplant process, he wasn't going to go along with it like a nodding dog, regretting his decision later.

Our hospital quickly suggested a second opinion within the NHS, so we met with a professor at Great Ormond Street who happened to be involved in a clinical drug trial we were on. To cut a long story short, he was kind but to the point and articulated that because Teddy was healthy, in remission and had a good stem cell donor match, he felt the transplant was the right thing to do. So, we agreed to go ahead with it.

Let's go to a question that isn't always easy to unpick. Once you are in the medical system – let's assume you are in the UK where we have the NHS – do you have the right to request a second opinion?

The General Medical Council, the governing body of doctors, state: "All doctors must respect the patient's right to seek a second opinion." The quality of the patient's care cannot be impacted by the request; however, patients do not have a legal right to receive one. If a doctor agrees that it could be in the patient's best interest to receive a second opinion, potentially due to limited experience with a rare condition, it will be recommended. NHS England will support a request for a second opinion in these circumstances. It is important to note that depending on your treatment plan and type of cancer this may require a referral via the GP, which could take time.

For a more urgent need for a second opinion in a hospital environment, a new initiative has recently been rolled out in the UK called Marsha's Rule following the death of a young child due to sepsis in circumstances that could have been potentially avoided. As a result, an independent rapid response team provides around the clock access if someone is concerned about someone's condition in hospital and there is a real risk to their life. Please seek more information online as the scope of these programmes can often change.

In round one of Teddy's treatments something happened which was the only time I was ever truly terrified for his safety. I'm telling you about it because it illustrates the importance of asking questions. I had swapped with Kurt as my mental health wasn't great after being isolated for almost five days because of a virus Ted's twin, George, might or might not have had. The initial shock of diagnosis had worn off, Ted was just a little under the weather, and I needed to get out of this tiny room that was suffocating me.

I was sobbing in the arms of a lovely nurse who we will call 'Phoebe' and a health care assistant – let's call Sally. Sally was my rock, and I was so happy whenever she was on shift for those six months we were in. She's gone on to study to be a nurse and any hospital she finds herself in will have no idea how lucky they are. Kurt came and swapped with me. Luckily for us, the hospital was only twenty-five minutes from home. So off I went home and did the usual mummy duty of painting on a smile for George, cuddling him and kissing him before settling him in bed and then having a glass of wine in the empty silence of a house not fully occupied. I sat in my bed, continuing to read and research till my eyes couldn't take anymore and I fell asleep.

I woke around two in the morning and of course, I checked my phone. A WhatsApp from Kurt said, "He's got a fever of forty and a heart rate of two hundred. I think they are really worried." You know what they say about flying: if you are worried in turbulence look at the cabin crew. If they aren't worried, don't be worried. I felt sick. We were obviously messaging back and forth and trying to call.

A heart rate of two hundred is really quite scary. Ted would usually have a heart rate of 116-120 when he was fever free and healthy or one hundred and forty with a fever. Of course, the next day I raced down there, and we swapped again. The fever went on for a few days but what was worse was the rash that slowly developed.

It was so bad that I couldn't show pictures of Teddy to my parents. I knew it would break them. I only showed my sister, and that photo still haunts me to this day. It was so bad that all the patches had almost joined together to look like someone had poured boiling water over him. They didn't have any answers, but I soon found out. This is why it is important to ask lots and lots of questions.

You have probably already gathered that I'm quite impatient. Teddy wasn't recovering from the rash as quickly as I hoped so I reached out in desperation to my oncology community. I won't need to change these names because they are and were such an incredible support system. There was Vicky, whose daughter (three months younger than Teddy) who had been diagnosed with AML some time before us. I met her in a Facebook group, and she had given me advice on the clinical trial we ended up joining. There was also Claire, who had actually been a customer of mine in my natural canine nutrition and supplement business. These mums were the first to help me identify that all might not be what it seemed with this rash.

Claire's advice was to get a full list of all the drugs and chemo's that Ted had been on, then to go online to a reputable website, ideally belonging to a governing body, and go through each and every one and look not only at common side effects but rare ones too. I sent Vicky the photo and told her that I thought it was a drug reaction. The first thing I think she said was, "Hold on, I need to ring you. That rash is the exact same thing that happened to my friend's son." When she sent me a photo of her friend's child, my jaw just fell to the floor. It wasn't easy to convince the medical team, though. Even with the photos.

And then it happened. On their wild goose chase of trying to find out what was causing Ted's fever and rash, it was decided that a CT scan was the next course of action. My biggest concern was how to get an eighteen-month-old to lie still and not kick off and scream. The suggestion was made for an antihistamine to be given to make him a little drowsy, which we did twenty mins prior. I can't tell you how long after we came back from the CT scan that it suddenly clicked. The rash was going – *really* going… it was almost gone.

There I was ferociously pressing the nurse call buzzer and demanding to see the doctor before handover. I explained to the nurse how important it was that the doctor came when she could. She had seen Teddy before, so I wanted her to see the change. It took three requests and several hours before she arrived by which point my blood was boiling. She and I had already had a run-in before when she suggested oramorph for Teddy's teething pain rather than paracetamol. I don't like drugs when they aren't needed. I can count on one hand the number of paracetamols I've had in my adult life. We made up later, but no one was going to tell me what I knew was best for my child. First rule of a good paediatrician, always listen to the mother's gut instinct. It doesn't mean you have to agree.

I told her in no uncertain terms that I expected to see our haematologist consultant at ward round in the morning. She was very non-committal and responded by saying it might or might not be drug induced. I was clear that if they didn't get our consultant to attend, they would not have my permission to administer any more antibiotics or other meds that they were trying.

The next day, Elizabeth, our haematologist, came in with the doctor. At this point I was tired, stressed, anxious and frankly helpless, and the lioness inside me was swinging her claws at anyone in her path.

"Something you are giving him is making him sick. Here's the list of drugs it could be, so until you can work it out, he's not having them," I said.

Elizabeth did the classic thing that many doctors do when they know I might be right. "Well, we have been on this plan for almost seven days so ok, let's try something new."

They did. And Ted recovered fast. The most painful part was six months later when I had the courage to read all the discharge letters. I read, "Drug-induced reaction in round one of chemo."

I still don't think I am over that. To see it confirmed in a formal letter damaged the trust I had in the team a little. It wouldn't have been difficult to have discussed it in person and apologised that I had felt unheard.

Moral of the story: Antihistamines will reduce symptoms in reactions but not in a virus.

This was the most dramatic scenario, but there were many more times I challenged doctors on their proposals for Teddy's treatment that had nothing to do with his front-line chemotherapy.

After you have a round of chemotherapy, the body's bone marrow, which produces blood cells, can be affected. This can lead to a drop in the levels of various types of blood cells, including red blood cells (which carry oxygen), white blood cells (which help fight infections) and platelets (which help with clotting). This drop in blood cell levels can result in anaemia, increased risk of infections and bleeding problems. When the bone marrow recovers, typically after a few weeks, the blood cell counts start to increase again, restoring the body's ability to function properly.

Neutrophils are a type of white blood cell that play a crucial role in the body's immune system. They act as the first line of defence against infections, quickly moving to sites of infection to destroy bacteria and other foreign bodies. Think of them as the body's 'frontline soldiers' that help keep you healthy by fighting off germs and preventing infections from taking hold.

Every time Teddy's body bounced back after chemo and his neutrophils came back up, he had a fever. I have no idea why. Every single time it meant going straight on antibiotics and a trip to our shared care hospital, which is where you have to go if you are back at home and your oncology child becomes unwell or has a temperature of thirty-eight or above.

Antibiotics are great in life-saving situations like sepsis, but they also destroy your gut health by taking away the good bacteria as well as the bad. Then there's the risk of antibiotic resistance. Some of the antibiotics they wanted to give Teddy in our shared care hospital had a risk of long-term damage to the kidneys or even deafness. Whilst I rarely convinced medics not to administer antibiotics, there were times when we were further out from transplant that I questioned and then negotiated for Teddy to receive a different type of antibiotic with less risk of long-term side effects. This usually happened when Teddy's nose was running like a tap and my whole house was full of your standard winter cold and our very experienced oncologist consultant was able to make a pragmatic risk assessment.

Many of those discussions where I challenged were done from a place of partnership and mutual respect. I would like to stress that I don't know how the oncologist doctors and nurses do what they do. I would be a daily sobbing mess, and, in the UK, they do that on nowhere near the pay they deserve. Try to choose your battles and hold your ground in a respectful tone and approach.

The senior doctor, Richard, in charge of the ward in the immediate period after Teddy got his magic donor cells (as we call them) wanted to send Teddy for a CT scan. Ted had spiked a fever, and the doctor felt it wasn't related to his neutrophils coming back. I was sure it was. He probably felt that way because of all the guidelines and check boxes they have to follow. I politely communicated that given the fact we were in full isolation due to him being so high risk and immunocompromised, I didn't feel comfortable with him being carted across a hospital alongside members of the public to have a scan in an uncontrolled environment. He agreed.

About five mins after that discussion, the nurse came in with the bloods slip to say the neutrophils were coming back. It meant the transplant was doing what it should, albeit a bit early. I still smile about that today. I think I said quietly and softly to Richard, "Too early, is it?" Whilst I think I irritated the hell out of a lot of doctors, I was always polite, and when I held tight to my views it was usually for something that turned out to be true.

With your conversations, try to understand the rationale. If you have concerns, raise them and ask, "I'm concerned about X… how can we reduce the risk?" If someone says there is no risk or dismisses your fears, you need to decide if it is a battle you want to take on. There is nothing worse than a life filled with regrets and I have very few regrets about Ted's journey and the battles I took on and confrontations I had.

There are other areas in which I actively suggest you appropriately challenge and question. The main one for us was about bringing food in for Teddy. When Teddy was first transferred to our main oncology hospital my husband stayed the night with him and called me to say that they were offering him Coco Pops for breakfast. I saw red and was shocked that the hospital would even offer an ultra-processed food to such a sick child. In hindsight, I understand that some children may only eat ultra-processed foods but nevertheless I was still angry and decided in that moment that with the exception of breakfast every meal Teddy ate would come from home. I recognise that I am coming from a place of privilege as our hospital was only a short drive from home; however, they still tried to stop me bringing in food and this is where the lioness really made her first appearance.

I remember marching down the ward with my food thermos in hand at such a ridiculous speed I might as well have been running. I wanted his food to stay as warm as possible and I was desperate for my child to eat and eat a meal that would make him happy because food isn't just about fuel, it's a whole experience and it should be enjoyable.

I knew the nurses were all looking at me from their station. I knew that someone was about to follow me into Teddy's room and tell me off or tell me he couldn't eat my food. But I wasn't going to listen so when the door did open and someone came, as predicted, to tell me that I couldn't feed Teddy food from outside, they received the following response: "Your food is garbage. I wouldn't feed that to my dog let alone a child going through cancer. Regardless, Teddy isn't eating what you are offering him and he needs to eat, so you aren't going to tell me how I can and can't feed my child." Harsh, I know, and I'm sorry, but at this point it was only two weeks since we got Teddy's devastating diagnosis and he was in his third hospital, all of which I had brought my food into. The nurse was just doing her job. I did apologise and I wasn't proud of myself, but I wasn't going to give in on this subject.

At a later time, a meeting with the deputy matron and the dietician went round in circles. I did offer other options, none of which they wanted to compromise on. I even offered to bring in my own pots and pans and cook in the parents' kitchen. They declined saying the parents' kitchen wasn't clean enough. So, we were at a stalemate. Eventually, we agreed that I could bring Teddy's food in as long as it was piping hot, and I could evidence the temperature. It had to be freshly cooked not reheated. I think they also talked about me signing something, obviously an insurance thing of sorts, but I never got it.

I bought a cheap meat thermometer from the supermarket that night and every time Teddy's lunch and dinner arrived, I grabbed the first nurse I could see to witness the temperature. If they weren't around, I took a photograph on my phone as evidence.

Hot food in a thermos typically loses heat at about 0.5-1 degree Celsius per hour. This can vary based on factors like the surrounding temperature, the initial temperature of the food, and the insulation quality of the thermos. It's important to note that these are rough estimates, and the actual rate of heat loss can vary. It's always a good practice to test your thermos with hot water first to gauge its insulation capabilities. If you pack the thermos to the brim, there's no air space which could contribute to the meal cooling down quicker.

I think it was because of these disputes in the early days, and the fact that Teddy was not a beige processed food eater, that I managed to have the hospital cook to my recipes during transplant. This was justifiable, given they had a hospital kitchen on our ward. During short stays it was just accepted that I would bring food from home. The key thing was, it didn't feel right to me that I couldn't bring in food where they were unable to meet his needs, so I questioned, and I questioned, and I asked for written copies of policies and never took anyone's word for it until I got the outcome I wanted.

To conclude this chapter, I want to acknowledge that sometimes things do go wrong and there are scenarios where there might be a need to involve an independent complaints body. In the UK it's called PALS. PALS stands for Patient Advice and Liaison Service. They are there to help patients, their families and carers with any concerns, questions or complaints they have about the National Health Service (NHS) care they receive. PALS provides support, information and advice on health services and can help to resolve issues or complaints informally.

If you live outside the UK, I may have a similar organisation under a different name to act as a bridge between patients and healthcare providers and ensure that patient concerns are heard and addressed effectively.

PALS primarily focuses on hospital care within the NHS, but they also cover other healthcare services like clinics and community health services. To contact PALS, you can usually find their contact details in hospitals, GP surgeries, and on the NHS website. You can call, email, or visit them in person to discuss any concerns or feedback you may have about your healthcare experiences. They are there to help and support you in navigating the healthcare system and addressing any issues you may encounter. I hope you never need them but know that they are there.

CHAPTER 10

NG AND PEG TUBE FEEDING

"In seeking truth you have to get both sides of a story."

- Walter Cronkite

Depending on the type of cancer or treatment someone has, an NG tube or a PEG tube might be recommended to support them in terms of taking medication or receiving synthetic feeds.

A nasogastric tube, (NG tube) is inserted through the nose and down the throat into the stomach. It is a more temporary solution and has to be changed out every four to twelve weeks depending on the tube type used by the hospital. It is most commonly used for administering medication to young children who aren't always the most willing to take medications and for giving synthetic milk feeds.

A stomach PEG – or percutaneous endoscopic gastrostomy – tube is a longer-term solution and is inserted directly through the abdominal wall into the stomach under general anaesthetic.

In this chapter, I want to share my experiences of both the NG and the PEG and explain why, if I knew then what I know now, I might not have resisted the NG so hard in the early days of diagnosis and how it could have helped us even more with our holistic approach of supporting his body and helping it in overcoming his disease.

Either an NG or a PEG tube could be recommended at the start of treatment based on known side effects of the treatment plan or during treatment as a result of someone struggling with appetite or a condition called mucositis, which can be incredibly painful and debilitating.

Mucositis is an inflammatory condition of the GI tract which runs from your mouth and throat, through your stomach and right down into your bottom. It can cause sores and lesions and is said to be a common side effect of chemotherapy and radiotherapy.

We were very lucky that Teddy never got mucositis. However, he did have an NG tube and a PEG. We actually fought for him to have the latter inserted just before his bone marrow transplant.

An NG tube, whilst a temporary measure, is usually pretty traumatic to have inserted, especially for young children who often have to be held down whilst the thin long tube is inserted down the throat via their nose. Luckily, the process lasts only a few seconds, usually with an experienced nurse performing the procedure. It is just one of the awful things that parents have to stand back and allow to happen to their child during treatment, but it can have some real benefits.

Teddy was first diagnosed in our local hospital, and we were quickly transferred to one of the best surgical hospitals in the country, which happened to be close to home. There, Teddy had a bone marrow test to assess the gene types of his disease and also have a Hickman line inserted. We covered this a little in Chapter 5. Whilst we were there, we met some of the doctors who worked at the oncology hospital which would become Teddy's primary care hospital. It was standard practice for the consultants to visit some of the newly diagnosed parents to set some expectations about the horrors that lay ahead before they were transferred to the oncology hospital.

Sonny was one of the doctors who came to see us, if memory serves. We still see him now. Great doctor, so friendly and warm and pragmatic. But I will be honest that I was like a deer in the headlights at that early point and felt like my head was somewhere up in the clouds, my feet hovering a few feet above the earth. It might not have been him. It was a bit like that feeling when you are still intoxicated from the night before and not in a good way. Teddy hadn't started on chemo yet, but they had started a medication to try and flush out some of the nasties and my child resembled Chunk out of *The Goonies*. Out of all the photos I have of Ted during treatment, those still bring me to tears. He didn't look like my child. He looked like the elephant man.

When Sonny and another doctor (let's call her Marie) came in to see us, I was in full 'rage at the world' mode. I felt sorry for myself: why me, why my family? I had eaten healthily during my pregnancy, cared well for my child and nurtured him and I had already lost too many friends and family to cancer. Wasn't it someone else's turn?

"You know he's going to need an NG tube?" Sonny said.

"Sorry, what's an NG tube?"

So, they went on to explain. That's when the reality hit me that very soon, I was going to have a bald, sick little baby with the telltale sign of cancer stuck to his face with a plaster for the world to see. I'm ashamed to say it but at that moment I felt embarrassed. I didn't want the world to see my child and know he was sick, not that I am sure who or where I thought he would see these imaginary people. I wanted to fly under the radar and treat cancer like a dirty little secret and come out the other side without anyone knowing. Don't ask me why I felt that way. This is just me being honest.

I think it's important to recognise that a cancer diagnosis can feel like a bereavement, and you can feel all of those strong emotions that come with grief. Anger, despair, denial, disbelief, shock and intense sadness. Don't judge yourself too harshly for the slightly less than perfect thoughts and feelings that crop up. It is a huge shock for all of us. It doesn't make us bad people; we just desperately want it to go away.

"No, he's not," I replied. "He won't need it."

They went on to say that he would almost certainly get mucositis due to the types of chemo he would receive for his type of leukaemia, and he would struggle to eat. I refused the tube being inserted that day, saying we would cross that bridge when we came to it. When they left, I spent all night researching mucositis and natural remedies to try and prevent it, which came up with suggestions like slippery elm powder, marshmallow root tea and supplements like L-glutamine and zinc.

After Teddy's first round of chemotherapy, he needed a bone marrow test under general anaesthetic to see whether the chemotherapy had successfully put Teddy's cancer into remission. It had, thank God: zero cancerous cells detected. It was as part of the preparation for that surgery that the subject of an NG tube came up again.

We had trained Teddy to take medication like a little birdy opening up his mouth without complaints and he was eating well and was healthy, with the exception of that hideous drug reaction I talked about in Chapter 9. The team were not giving up on the fact that they felt he needed an NG tube despite the fact that all the evidence still suggested he didn't need it. At that point, Teddy was running around the ward like a mini tornado, stealing the nurse's trolleys and taking them for a spin up and down the corridors. I had now spoken about tubes to more mums in the know who had children with complex medical conditions that weren't cancer, and I was feeling more anti-NG tube and the trauma I felt Ted would regularly go through having it inserted, but as I mentioned there was information lacking at that time that would have swung in its favour.

But I was exhausted at this point. I had just had the supplement fight with our dietician, and I didn't feel like I could fight much more, and I wanted a break. I knew, however, that this NG wasn't going to work. My strong, rambunctious, healthy little toddler was not going to accept a piece of plastic hanging in the back of his throat. I remember telling our dietician that I would give it less than a day before Ted pulled it out, but I would allow them to try as it would be under a general anaesthetic (GA), and he wouldn't feel a thing.

It lasted less than an hour. We were back on the ward. Ted was recovering from the effects of his GA and was sat up eating his beloved organic rice cakes. Lisa, our dietician, was in the room and commented on how good it was that Teddy was eating a hard food with the NG tube fitted given it was such a new thing for him. We turned to have a conversation with one of the lovely health care assistants about something else which I swear lasted a few seconds. When we turned back, the NG lay next to him, face plaster and all. Internally, I was laughing so hard. I thought to myself, "Ok, baby, I hear you, just like your mummy. You don't want it, so you aren't having it." An NG tube never lasted more than a few days without this child pulling it out, sometimes with real force.

In one of my many conversations with our dietician, it suddenly came up that I could use the NG tube to administer juices, herbal teas and vegetable broths into Teddy. Some time had passed in terms of our treatment journey, and I remember thinking, "Given that you know about my nutrition ambitions and how I want to support Teddy, why have you taken so long to tell me this?" The advice was simple. Broths and juices were fine, but no thick soups or blended meals and they advised against anything sticky like a meat stock that could block the tube. I also had to make sure I gave it a good flush afterwards with warm, not hot water. I thought that was pretty reasonable and this was a huge help when Teddy spent seven days in hospital when he got a line infection (and technically sepsis) due to negligence.

I mentioned earlier that when the subject of an NG tube came up, I sought advice from people outside of the oncology community who were using tubes with their children with medically complex needs. I was so lucky to have my friend Kim as one of these people to guide me. Kim and I originally met in my canine nutrition and wellness group on Facebook, linked to my online natural supplements shop. Kim is mother to a child with medically complex needs and her daughter Lillie has a permanent version of the stomach PEG as she cannot receive food orally.

Kim would often share, even before Teddy was diagnosed, these wonderful meals that she would make and blend for Lillie and then administer through her gastric tube. Kim also had experience with NG tubes as her own dad had one during his cancer treatment. If anyone knew anything about getting good nutrition into the body in the absence of being able to eat orally, I knew it would be Kim. I also knew she had the same values on nutrition as I did.

Kim is and was a huge advocate for blended diets and had even been involved in studies in her local area and hospital to evidence the benefits for children who need support with feeding. Her advice to me was very clear: push for a peg so you can achieve your goals, and she told me which books to buy and areas to research.

Prior to having a bone marrow transplant, the patient (or their legal guardians if under the age of eighteen) has to go through a number of meetings to sign a consent form for the transplant to go ahead. I think it is to ensure it is an *informed* consent and that you understand all the risks and procedures, because fundamentally there's at minimum a ten percent risk of death as a result of the transplant.

I went alone to one of those meetings later during the process, although I can't remember exactly why. In the meeting were our transplant consultant, our transplant clinical nurse specialist, Lisa our dietician and me. We knew all the key information about the donor we were using, and we were looking into fertility preservation and some of the more intricate details about the admission. I had already emailed with Lisa several times to share my desire for Teddy to have a PEG tube and a blended diet administered should he stop eating. I even offered to buy an expensive Thermomix so I could cook in our hospital room and blend it myself so I could feed him via the PEG tube. I had hoped that the hospital's infection control department would approve it as a Thermomix is a self-contained multi cooker and kitchen device.

During the meeting, I told our transplant consultant that I wanted Teddy to have a PEG fitted. I was aware of a study taking place at the leading UK children's hospital on the benefits of a PEG during transplant, led by a man called James Evans. A paper published online in 2021 had indicated that having a PEG tube could improve quality of life for Teddy during transplant and reduce the risk of him needing to have TPN, which is like a complete nutrition IV bypassing the gut system. Being a big believer in the power of the gut system and the microbiome for immunity and remaining strong during cancer treatment, I wanted to keep Teddy's gut moving at all costs. The transplant consultant wasn't keen, but Lisa supported the insertion of a PEG given the number of NG tube replacements Teddy had already had.

It was agreed that as long as he was fit and well for surgery, he would have a PEG inserted at the surgical hospital a month prior to treatment but they made it clear that they wouldn't be willing to delay our transplant date because of it. Luckily for us, it all worked out well. Teddy had the PEG fitted in July 2022.

Lisa and I had many power struggles during my time in treatment and whilst I was willing to stop at nothing to advocate for my child in what I felt was a better and more natural way, I do respect what she was trying to do and how she was trying to help based on the limitations placed on her by the health care system. She surprised me when she shared in a meeting that she had advocated for Teddy to be allowed to have baby pouches administered through his PEG tube should it be required. She had gone to a national board to state his case as I was hell bent on saying that if Teddy wouldn't eat the meals that the hospital had agreed to cook to my recipes, then those meals should be blended so I could put them down the peg. Infection control had refused this request based on the risk of using a blender and contamination risks which to this day I really don't understand.

Teddy was only the second child in the whole of the UK approved for individual baby pouches to be fed down the PEG and this was instrumental in the two weeks post-transplant when Teddy had days, he didn't want to eat but I could keep his gut nourished with goodness. That was all her doing. I can take no credit for it.

Teddy flew through his transplant requiring no TPN, no pain medication, no milk feeds and no complications. This is unheard of, and I am sure that without the PEG this would not have been possible. Teddy had it removed five months post-transplant and is left with a small scar like a second indented belly button. They weren't able to do a full reversal as the initial procedure meant his stomach was attached to his abdomen, which they can't remove but is not expected to cause him any long-term issues. It was a price worth paying for how well he did through such a horrific procedure. I am very grateful to Lisa for helping me achieve those goals and I hope that in the future it will influence hospitals' thinking for other children and adults going through transplant. Not only are drugs like TPN incredibly expensive for the healthcare system, but they also significantly delay a child's return to normal eating and impact quality of life.

CHAPTER 11

TEDDY'S PLAN... EXACTLY AS WE DID IT

This chapter gives you Teddy's exact support plan and recipes for the period when he was going through chemotherapy and also post-transplant.

What I share with you is not a substitute for medical advice and I stress the importance of working with your or your loved one's oncology team in partnership and being completely open and honest about what you are doing. Whilst they will tell you 'We do not recommend' supplements or have less faith than I do in the power of food to support a body going through cancer treatment, we do want to keep everyone safe.

If they say that there is evidence that a supplement is unsafe and proven unsafe against a medication that's being taken, please do not ignore it.

Use my plans by way of ideas you can research using reputable sources such as the websites PubMed and NIH and then take to your team to discuss.

PubMed is a free online tool run by a government organisation called the National Institute of Health. It is pretty up to date with the newest research and the information comes from highly respected science journals. Search on PubMed using the key words IP6, and leukaemia and you will see some of the incredible and mind-blowing research that really should be more widely known in mainstream medicine. This particular article talks about the potential of IP6 to cause leukaemia cells to commit apoptosis (cell suicide). The one about effects of blueberry extracts on AML leukaemia was also a pretty mind-blowing read.

Your team may have concerns about their inability to recommend supplements due to restrictions placed upon them by the system they operate in, but I want you to come from a place of being able to make an informed decision for the journey which I hope will lead to remission and ultimately cure.

Before discussing with your team, I also recommend you check online for known drug interactions with supplements. It is always best to go into your meetings as fully informed as possible to avoid emotional distress as a result of being challenged or not getting the response you want. I always remember talking to our haematologist consultant in the early days about the research I had found on wild blueberries and the studies with AML. I felt excited that I believed I had found something which could help Teddy and then felt flat when I got zero reaction or emotion from her. I regularly used the website **https://naturalmedicines.therapeuticresearch.com/** to check for drug and supplement interactions. I paid for a yearly subscription to the site, but there are other, free ways to do this. I didn't have the patience and wanted instantaneous answers.

When the hospital claimed there was a potential risk of side effects of certain supplements, what worked for me was understanding what the likelihood was, what the risk looked like and also what the fix would be. As an example, if they said there could be a risk (that they couldn't quantify) that it could impact Teddy's platelets. The fix would be to give him platelets. I took the risk, but he never needed additional platelets due to taking supplements. There were also risks of the traditional medicines having side effects but not doing those is rarely an option.

Whilst I created most of Teddy's plan myself, I worked with herbalists and our naturopathic doctor Kate James within a month of Teddy being diagnosed, who gave me the foundation and recommended supplements I hadn't heard of before (like IP6) that were game changing. I made sure I had the right people to soundboard with, in a professional capacity so that I wouldn't be giving him too many supplements. This isn't great for the body as it has to process the excess out and also can lead to burnout and overwhelm for the patient or caregiver trying to administer.

One of the most common questions I get asked on social media is whether or not this plan is suitable for patients who have a different type of cancer and not leukaemia. The answer is yes, with the disclaimer that I have never made the claim that our plan cured Teddy's cancer but that I believe it helped support his body to fight cancer alongside conventional treatment. It kept his body strong and his vital vitamin and mineral levels up while treatments by design would deplete them. I opted for all-natural food-based supplements as much as possible, which means they were made one hundred percent from food, no additives and no fillers. The exception to this was the vitamin D3+ K2. That was a synthetic supplement, but I chose a brand I trusted that transpired to have been set up following the founder's cancer journey. I have had people contact me from all over the world, from the UK where we live and in the United States and Australia, all of whom are using our method having seen our journey on social media to great success with the backing and support of their medical teams.

A final note before I give you our step-by-step plan and a few recipes: you will notice that Teddy's plan changed after his bone marrow (stem cell) transplant. This is because I have never stopped learning about nutrition and natural remedies, not for one day since the day he was diagnosed on 1st April 2022. My undiagnosed ADHD meant I would survive in hospital on less than four hours of sleep, learning about different herbs and proactively taking more courses on the gut microbiome and the link with our gut and the immune system. I was so desperate to find a magic bullet that would see him through treatment safely and reduce his risk of relapse that I couldn't stop looking. I now know even more certainly than before that there isn't a single thing – it's about supporting the body with a wider variety of things. That's where I truly believe the magic lies in better outcomes and fewer long-term side effects for cancer patients.

TEDDY'S PLAN – KEY NUTRITION PRINCIPLES

(Again, this is just a guide)

Focus on the good not the bad: Choosing to take a holistic approach and focus on nutrition can feel overwhelming. However, my best advice would be to focus on getting good healthy nutrition and whole foods and plants into the diet rather than being obsessed about eating a single rich tea biscuit. At home, we use a tracker I made which I want to give you as a free PDF resource. Make it fun and it will make the whole process feel so much less overwhelming. You can find the free resource on my website:

www.cancerisntallaboutchemo.com

No cold foods: Warm meals *only*. This is based on a traditional Chinese medicine principle that when the body is already under strain and stress you shouldn't make the digestive system work harder by breaking down uncooked food. Teddy didn't eat sandwiches or raw salad produce, although he did have fruit, especially berries, and he loved bananas which are a rich source of potassium.

Drinks: No cold water. Room temperature water only and focus on warm herbal teas or plant based organic milk alternatives.

Minimal dairy: I'm not a fan of dairy but I won't focus on it because it can be controversial. Teddy was drinking cows' milk when he was diagnosed but I quickly switched him to an organic oat milk. I personally feel that where I live milk is highly processed. Most livestock are overly pumped with antibiotics and my mother raised me as a child to avoid dairy when I had a cold or was unwell. So, we cut it out but I did allow Teddy to have some pretty junky yoghurts so I could hide supplement powders in them. You choose your battles.

No more than four ingredients in foods that aren't homemade: Learn to read the labels of what you choose to eat or feed your loved one. If there is an ingredient you cannot pronounce or buy to cook with yourself, avoid it if at all possible.

Cooking oils: Best oils for a high smoke point are ghee, avocado oil and coconut oil. I like coconut oil for gut health. Use tallow for things like homemade chips or roast potatoes and if you want to use olive oil, add it towards the end of your cooking. Sauté onions in a drop of water instead if not using coconut oil or ghee. Some products that you wouldn't expect have rapeseed oil hidden in them. I'm not a fan and won't touch it but do your own research.

No pasteurised products: During treatment our team didn't want me to use raw honey or manuka, so I switched to organic maple syrup. The honey that was 'allowed' is highly processed with none of the natural benefits you find in real honey.

Fish and meat – quality over quantity: Wild caught salmon over organic or farmed salmon. Organic grass-fed meat where budget allows. When our budgets were tight, we made meat go further by bulking it out with vegetables, beans and legumes.

Teddy's Pre-transplant Supplement Regime

- IP6 and Inositol, three times a day mixed in a drink. Ideally, on an empty stomach.
- Zinc
- Blue green algae
- Coq10 – will need a break on days leading up to chemo and a few days thereafter.
- Liposomal vitamin C
- Vitamin D3+K2
- High quality fish oil (choose a brand that tests for heavy metals)
- Loov Wild Blueberry Powder
- Lucuma powder

Teddy's Post-Transplant Regime

- IP6 three times a day till twelve months post-transplant
- Elderberry syrup from autumn until spring
- Black seeds oil two or three times per week
- Fish oil
- Vitamin D3+K2
- Liposomal vitamin C
- Chaga mushroom powder
- Reishi mushroom powder
- Lion's mane mushroom powder
- Blue green algae

Drinks

- Coconut water – add in some fresh fruit if needed. Great for hydration.
- Chamomile tea – organic tea bags from the supermarket.
- Fennel tea – organic tea bags or boil some fresh fennel. Great for digestion.
- Medical Medium's mushroom healing broth - See medical mediums website for full recipe.

—RECIPES—

DRINKS

Golden milk

Ingredients

2 cups plant-based milk (oat, almond or coconut are recommended)
1 tsp ground turmeric
½ tsp ground cinnamon
½ tsp ground ginger or 1 tsp fresh ginger
Pinch black pepper
Maple Syrup - to taste

Method

In a small saucepan combine the plant-based milk, turmeric, ginger, cinnamon and black pepper. Whisk the mixture to ensure spices are well distributed.
Heat the mixture on a medium heat, mixing frequently until warm. Do not bring to a boil.

Miracle ABC Juice

Ingredients

1 apple
2 medium beetroots
3 carrots
1 small piece of ginger (optional)

Method

Wash your ingredients with a clean brush under running water. Chop apples and beetroots in half of quarters based on your juicer's requirements. Feed all the ingredients through your juicer. Pour juice into glass and serve, consuming within 20 minutes for the most benefit.
Notes - Use organic ingredients where possible to access the most benefits from the skin of the ingredients. If you are using organic ingredients, you are still required to wash the ingredients prior to juicing.

BREAKFAST

Teddy's Magic Purple Porridge - Beginners

Please note this is an average child's single portion. For those with a greater appetite, increase the volume of oats and plant-based milk but you do not need to increase the volume of the other ingredients.

Ingredients

½ cup of organic gluten free organic oats
1 cup of plant-based milk
1/4 tsp Loov Wild Blueberry Powder or 1 tbsp wild blueberries
¼ tsp Naturya Organic Lucuma Powder
¼ tsp ground, ¼ tsp chia seeds, ¼ tsp hemp seeds
½ tsp maple syrup

Method

Add porridge oats and milk to the hob. Cook on a medium heat until the volume has reduced by 50%. Remove from the stove and put in the bowl. Add a little plant-based milk to ensure that consistency is not too thick and sticky. Add in wild blueberry powder, lucuma powder or choice of additional item and a drizzle maple syrup on top. Mix well and serve.

Teddy's Magic Purple Porridge - Advanced

Ingredients

½ cup of organic gluten free organic oats
1 cup of plant-based milk
1 tbsp cooked buckwheat or frozen cauliflower rice
¼ tsp Loov Wild Blueberry Powder or 1 tbsp wild blueberries
½ tsp raw organic bee pollen
1 tsp raw honey or manuka honey
1 tsp ground nuts and seeds, aim to include: walnuts, brazil nuts, pistachios, pumpkin seeds, chia seeds, flax seeds, hemp seeds
1 powdered dandelion capsule (open capsule and add to cooked porridge)
1 powdered burdock capsule (open capsule and add to cooked porridge)

Method

Add porridge oats and milk to a pan on the hob. Cook on a medium heat until the volume of milk has reduced by 50%. Add in your cooked buckwheat or cauliflower rice. Remove from the stove and add to the serving bowl. Add a little plant-based milk to ensure that consistency is not too thick and sticky. Add in wild blueberry powder, bee pollen, honey, seeds and contents of the capsules. Mix well and serve.

LUNCH OR DINNER

Aunty Eva's Lentil Soup

Ingredients

250g brown lentils
400g chopped tomatoes
1 medium carrot
2 litres filtered water
1 medium/large potato
1 onion
1 tsp extra virgin olive oil
1 tsp smoked paprika
1 tbsp corn flour

Method

Chop the carrots and potato into very small pieces, no larger than your small fingernail.
Chop onions finely. Add lentils, water and chopped tomatoes to the pan and cook on a high heat and then bring to a boil before simmering until all ingredients are soft. Can take between 45 minutes - 1 Hour.
Towards the end of the cooking time, take 1½ tbsp of fluid from the soup into a bowl, mix with flour to make a slurry and put back into soup to thicken. Allow the soup to cook for at least a further 5-10 minutes before serving.

Mediterranean Chicken Pesto Pasta

Ingredients

½ medium red onion
4 tsp sundried tomato pesto
1 tbsp avocado oil/ghee/coconut oil
1 pack organic skinless boneless chicken thighs
1 medium courgette
1 medium red bell pepper
3 garlic cloves
225g baby plum/cherry tomatoes
1 cup fresh basil
1 tbsp mixed herbs (Italian)
1 tbsp nutritional yeast
400g chopped tomatoes

Method

Marinate the chicken thighs in 2 tsp of pesto and place into the fridge for at least 30 minutes.
Preheat the oven. Place your chicken thighs on parchment paper and bake in the oven till ready.
Chop courgette and bell pepper into small cubes. Heat oil and sauté the pepper and courgette for 57 minutes. Add the chopped tomatoes, basil nutritional yeast, garlic and basil and simmer. Remove chicken from the oven and cut into smaller pieces. Add the chicken to the pan and mix well. Add nutritional yeast, 2 tsp pesto and cook for a further 10 minutes or until courgettes are edible but not too soft.
Notes - Serve with brown rice fusilli pasta, wholewheat pasta, chickpea pasta or lentil pasta.

Chuck It All in Curry

Ingredients

1 onion
2 small carrots
4 chicken thighs
Madras curry paste
Firm tofu
1 red bell pepper
140g firm tofu
500g chopped tomatoes
1 cup shiitake mushrooms, stems removed
4 crushed garlic cloves
1 cup tender stem broccoli
1 cup chopped green beans
2 cups spinach (chopped)
1 tablespoon coconut oil/avocado oil/ghee

Method

Marinate chicken thighs in madras curry paste and place in the fridge for at least 30 minutes. For reduced spice levels use ½ of the paste.
Chop all ingredients finely including tender stems – do not throw stalks away this is where all the nutrients are.
Sauté onion and carrots in oil. Cut chicken thighs into small bite size chunks. Sear in the same pan as onions and carrots and add in chopped tomatoes, bell pepper, green beans and tofu.
Put on a high heat and simmer until chicken is almost fully cooked.
Add shiitake mushrooms, garlic and spinach 10 minutes before the end of cooking.
Notes - Serve with brown basmati rice.

Mumma's Supercharged Spaghetti

Ingredients

1kg grass fed beef mince
300ml of veg broth or bone broth
1 onion
1 medium sized carrot
1 medium celery stalk
8 cloves of garlic
2 organic chopped tomatoes
½ tsp dried rosemary.
1 tbsp of Worcestershire sauce
1 cup of shiitake mushrooms finely chopped
100g chopped fresh basil
1 tablespoon tomato puree
2 tsp dried oregano
1 tbsp ghee/avocado oil
1 tsp extra virgin olive oil
Celtic sea salt and pepper to season

Method

Finely chop the onion, celery, and carrots. Add oil to a warm pan with oil. Add the celery onion and carrots and sauté for 5 minutes until onions are translucent. Brown the beef and add the rosemary, tomato puree. Cook for 5-10 minutes.

Add chopped tomatoes, Worcestershire sauce and mix well for a further 5-10 minutes. Add the vegetable stock and shiitake mushrooms and cook until the volume of liquid has almost halved.

Add olive oil and fresh basil, oregano and garlic as the liquid begins to reduce and can be seen on the side of the pan.

Notes – Add herb amounts based on personal preferences. Oregano has a stronger taste than basil so a 1:2 ratio is recommended. Serve with brown pasta, wholewheat or lentil pasta.

CHAPTER 12

DETOX

"Detoxing is not a punishment. It's a celebration of your body and its ability to heal."

- Unknown

This chapter is about life after treatment and for those who have a level of health anxiety about getting cancer and want to do a little extra than just 'live a healthy lifestyle'.

Whilst I use the word detox throughout this chapter because it's a term that resonates with people the most, the process that I am about to describe to you is so much more than that. I will try to avoid the cliché of calling it a lifestyle change but what we did for Teddy post-treatment was with the intention of putting his body back into balance after receiving incredibly aggressive chemo, transplant drugs and all the other pharmaceuticals that live in the margins of an oncology journey.

Homeostasis is the medical/scientific term used for balance within the body. The words come from two Greek words meaning *stability*, and this is what I wanted to create for Teddy and his future. Stability. Stability for a future in spite of the risk of secondary cancers as a result of treatment. We know that if you have had cancer once and have had conventional treatment for cancer you do have a statistical risk of being diagnosed with a secondary cancer not associated with your initial diagnosis.

I will never judge anyone who chooses to walk away after treatment and live a life as if cancer never happened to them and to not make any lifestyle changes, but for me it didn't sit right. With Teddy being such a young child when he was diagnosed, I felt it my duty to try and safeguard his future as much as possible so he could go on and live a long and happy life. I just pray the efforts we have put in at such an early-stage post-treatment will support his body and afford him a level of protection. Sometimes I feel every way I turn I see people struggling with chronic illnesses, largely due to conditions that can be traced back to chronic inflammation within the body.

I will take the opportunity here to say that what I am about to share with you is what I chose to do based upon information I read, how I interpreted it and what I felt was best for my family and our future. Your personal journey is yours and yours alone and I am under no circumstances saying you must do what I did for Teddy in terms of a detox. I am also, of course, not guaranteeing that this will mean you will never get a primary or secondary diagnosis, but I will guide you thus far: the principles I adopted are safe, well researched and backed by science.

They were also carried out under the eyes of the medical team who regularly performed blood tests on Ted, as is standard post-transplant, and also our naturopathic doctor, Kate. If you are under the care of a doctor for any reason, I stress that you should share your intentions with them.

Now that the introductions are out of the way, let's talk about how I suggest you could get your body into a better state of balance, thereby detoxing it, mainly by supporting its natural detoxing process. I see a lot of comments online that detoxes are an unnecessary fad because the body naturally detoxes itself. I agree and disagree with this statement, and I will explain why. But before I do, I think the likely main reason people don't buy into detox is because the term has been overused to sell individual supplements or fad diets. From firsthand experience, I can tell you that detoxing the body and putting the body back into a state of balance takes time and dedication. It's not a five-day maple syrup and lemon water fast that I tried almost twenty years ago. Achieving balance within the body takes time.

A body that is healthy and adequately supported will naturally carry out a detoxification process. However, a body that has been under strain either through cancer treatment, poor diet, stress, large volumes of pharmaceutical medications or living in an unhealthy environment (such as a home with previous water damage and invisible mould) will struggle. Even if you haven't been through an oncology journey, I still feel there is incredible value in supporting your body and focusing on keeping it in balance so it can detox. There are so many outside influences that can have a negative impact on our bodies, from ultra-processed foods and the pressure to have a successful career whilst managing a family, to the environmental toxins we are exposed to like the pesticides on food and heavy metals in our day-to-day lives.

I think cultural norms have pushed us to such an extent that self-care looks like a bath with a face pack once a week or a night out with friends, rather than looking at how we can proactively keep our bodies strong by doing good things for it little and often. I am also guilty of these things, but we should never stop trying to invest in ourselves. As the saying goes, our health is our wealth.

There are several organs involved in the body's natural detoxification process and I will run through these with you now. The key organs are the liver, kidneys, lungs, skin and the digestive system. The liver is the star of the show as it takes harmful materials from the digestive tract and turns them into less harmful material to be excreted.

The kidneys filter the blood to remove excess substances and waste products. They produce urine to remove these products from the body, which is why water intake is so important prior to considering any detox.

Your lungs actually help remove some toxins simply by breathing.

Your skin is a barrier and whilst it also helps regulate body temperature you can push a small number of waste products and toxins out through it. This is why saunas are often referenced as a helpful tool in supporting the body's natural detox process and there is a lot of science out there that could support these claims. This is something I would certainly try as Ted gets older, having spent much of my time in Germany growing up in a sauna with my grandparents.

The gastrointestinal tract is the final key organ in the body's natural detoxing process. It breaks down food, absorbing the nutrients and pushing out waste products via bowel movements. This is why regular bowel movements are important. In my opinion once or twice a day is optimal… yes, even for children. If you go less, I recommend looking at increasing the fibre-rich whole foods within your diet and making sure you drink enough water.

Another key point I would like to make is if you choose to do more aggressive detox practices when your body isn't in a healthy state, you are at risk of having what's called a Herx reaction or die-off symptoms. Regardless of what some influencers might tell you online, I do not agree this is par for the course: I actually think it's dangerous. It signals you have tried to run before you can walk and your body is in distress.

A Herx reaction (Herxheimer to give it its full name) is an immune system reaction that occurs when a large volume of toxins is released into the bloodstream after the death of pathogens. Pathogens is an umbrella term for bacteria, viruses, fungi and parasites. It doesn't last long but can be deeply unpleasant, especially for those whose bodies have been through cancer treatment. It is also not necessary. Examples of a potential Herx reaction include, but are not limited to, flu-like symptoms, feeling lethargic, skin rashes, headaches, irritability, nausea and loose stools.

Let's now cover all the practices we did with Teddy to try and support his body's natural detoxification process. This is presented as a step plan, not because I am promoting you to follow it but because it is the easiest way to paint a picture of our journey.

Teddy had regular and good bowel movements throughout treatment and thereafter. Regular and good quality bowel movements are key, I think, because if you want the bad stuff out, the gut really needs to be helping get it out. The Bristol stool chart is a great tool to search online if you need further guidance about the quality of bowel movements.

Optimise nutrition, aiming for 35-50 plant materials a week, including vegetables, fruits, beans, legumes, nuts and seeds and fresh herbs. I have a basic workbook tracker that helped me track our numbers every week, ticking the foods off one by one. (I offer this tracker to others. You can find more information on this via my website.) It made meal planning fun because as a working mum with twin toddlers, trying to remember it all was overwhelming. I also share regular recipes on social media and have a recipe book which I offer to people, as I have made it my mission to hide more diversity into our diet without us even realising. I did this in basic meals like shepherd's pie and spaghetti bolognaise and our famous Teddy's magic purple porridge.

It also felt like a fun competition with me. I would sit down every Friday in my lunch break at work and look at the previous weeks to spot the areas where I had gaps so that at the end of each month, I would feel we were having real variety to feed those all-important healthy gut microbes. We aimed where we could for 150g of cruciferous vegetables daily for the children and 300g for the adults to support the liver so it could best perform its detoxification process. This was recommended to me by my own nutritionist mentor, Natalie, but you can get more support on this via my website.

I totally understand that this could feel overwhelming if you have been through cancer treatment and have experienced taste changes. I was there too, after transplant. Even though Teddy had always been a good eater, we had to start little by little. As an example, when I was adding a new item to his porridge such as a seed type, I started with ⅛ of a teaspoon and very slowly worked my way up. I would never try to add in more than one new thing a week. Two years post-transplant, he eats a daily porridge of organic oats, buckwheat, cauliflower rice, six types of nuts and seeds, with berries and all the adaptogenic mushroom powders thrown in, hidden with some natural raw honey and bee pollen. And he devours it every morning. Take your time and never put pressure on yourself or someone you love to accept changes overnight.

Anti-inflammatory foods are really important to the body, and not only if you have been on a cancer treatment journey. Examples are turmeric, garlic, fatty fish, berries, apples, green tea, and cruciferous vegetables like broccoli to name just a few.

They are so good because they support the lymphatic system. The lymphatic system is a crucial part of the body's immune system that is involved in supporting the removal of waste products, nutrient absorption and protecting against infections. Some of what we did for Ted, outside of his diet, was to do with supporting his body's lymphatic drainage process.

Looking to support your body's lymphatic drainage process, whether you have/had cancer or not, is important for a number of reasons outside of detox. For one, it is said to support the body's lymphatic function and by doing so supports the body's ability to identify and attack abnormal cells, which could be cancerous cells. It also is said to help promote the immune system's circulation of lymphocytes. Lymphocytes are the types of white blood cells essential for fighting infections and disease. This is probably why Teddys lymphocyte count was always really high whenever he had a common cold. Lymphatic drainage treatments or therapies can also be a great stress reducer and encourage calmness whilst promoting the healing process, which is ideal for those who have been through surgery.

I won't go into the different parts of the body that make up the lymphatic system, but I do want to mention that your tonsils and adenoids form a part of it. When we had to explore options for Teddy's glue ear, which was discovered a year after treatment, and grommets and a potential removal of his adenoids was recommended, it was a hard no from me. There wasn't any reason to, it was just suggested as a precaution.

Some people have to have lymph nodes remove as part of treatment, which is necessary due to their medical situation. For those people, I highly recommend finding a practitioner who specialises in lymphatic drainage massages as those individuals can struggle with oedema, which can be localised to involve significant fluid retention or can risk more serious conditions like liver and kidney disease. I had oedema in the later stage of my twin pregnancy, like many mums, and I ended up wearing my husband's size ten trainers immediately after I gave birth to be able to leave the house. I really feel for people who have to live with it on an ongoing basis.

A lot of the therapies recommended for lymphatic drainage can be difficult or impossible with a young child/toddler. Massage and acupuncture for us were just a no-go but something I will look to discuss with Teddy as he gets older. As you might have worked out, I have a big interest in traditional Chinese medicine, which acupuncture is a part of, and I actually had several sessions before we attempted to conceive in an attempt to get my body into balance before being pregnant.

For us, having researched the topic there was one thing that really stood out as being easy to do and having the least path of resistance whilst also working on his core body strength: that was rebounding (trampolining). Yes, bouncing up and down on a trampoline and releasing your inner child can have a really helpful impact on your lymphatic drainage system.

It's a low impact exercise compared to something like running. It can also help reduce stress and through its rhythmic up and down movement encourages the movement of lymph fluid throughout the body whilst also discouraging fluid from building in the tissues which may develop into oedema. We got Teddy a little toddler trampoline for our home and visited a local children's trampoline park when we were allowed out into the real-world post-transplant. Compared to his twin brother he wasn't enamoured with it, but it's a practice we can easily slot into our lives and it's good to know that it has hidden benefits for his body.

Another easy method to support the body's natural detoxification process that we implemented as soon as his

Hickman line was removed was to start doing gentle detox baths. These types of baths went viral for a time on social media due to claimed benefits for neurodivergent children or those with language delays and also for those who just needed to show their body a little extra love and support. We did them not with the view that they were going to detox Teddy of all the strong medications he had during treatment, but with the view that they were gentle, could support a calm and restful night's sleep, and if they supported his body in detoxing or getting over common winter viruses quicker, even better.

The baths consist of adding one or two cups of Epsom salts or magnesium flakes, a half to a full cup of bentonite clay and a half to one cup of baking soda. I tried one myself before using it on the boys and I have to say I slept incredibly well that evening. But magnesium does that to the body. It is one of the nutrients we deplete most quickly when we are stressed. You know all about the power of sleep from my earlier chapter so it felt like it could do no harm as long as I was only doing it a couple of nights a week and making sure the boys had plenty to drink afterwards as the baths encourage the body to sweat. But the boys enjoyed me not pressuring them to get them out of the bath, letting them play and pretend to be mermen. Can I say for sure that they aid detox? I can't... but I do know that sweating encourages the body's natural detoxification process and each bath cost pennies and had no risk of harm as they were neither pregnant nor had kidney issues.

Given the amount of time that cancer patients spent in bed, whether sitting or sleeping, we decided approximately eighteen months post-transplant and thereby the end of his treatment to start seeing an osteopath. For us our therapist practised in similar methods to a cranial chiropractor which is something becoming more popular for mothers with young children who have had c sections or traumatic births. Often referred to as craniosacral therapy, this type of therapy involves the gentle manipulation of the skull and spine but no clicking or cracking. Claimed benefits include improvement in sleep, reduced symptoms of colic and also supporting the central nervous system and reducing stress.

Kurt and I tried as much as possible not to treat Teddy like a sick child in treatment. We would keep him on his feet as much as possible, based on his energy levels and his ability each day. The oncology journey involves so much sitting or lying down and for us the quotes we had heard of 'use it or lose it' stuck in our minds. As a result, it made sense for us to see an osteopath post-treatment, or someone qualified in chiropractic's in children to try and unpick some of the physical tension in his body. Ted didn't mind the sessions as it meant some rare screen time and our therapist Sabrina was wonderful and so gentle and we saw some great gains in his core strength and motor skill development.

Supplement-wise, detox can look slightly different for many. Some people work on principles of trying to extract heavy metals from the body. For us, we continued in large with our post-transplant plan that you can find in Chapter 12, and I also did phases of different detox practices. This usually meant phases of focusing on looking at one type and giving the body time to realign itself before looking at something different. I believe in the power of diversity in the body. You can eat chicken and steamed broccoli every day, but I don't think that makes you particularly healthy; I think variety is key. So, we went through periods where I would offer Teddy and George a homemade celery juice first thing in the morning or lemon with warm water and ginger. Other times we would follow Medical Medium's heavy metal detox smoothie recipes. We were always mixing it up.

I have also explored the use of zeolites and binders to help detox the body and this is a path we are newly on. Zeolites are a mineral that claim to attract and absorb heavy metals found within the body and, like a magnet, collect them and push them out of the body through excretion. This is done through a process called ion exchange.

You have to do a lot of research as some companies out there offer zeolite products that are better than others. However, Teddy is showing some developmental gains, and they are pretty simple to use and aren't particularly taxing financially.

But, as with all things, I believe you need a good foundation of putting the good things into the body first before trying to take away the bad. It is the same principle as the one I apply to nutrition.

Apple pectin's are currently an area of interest that I am researching due to claims of being radiation protective. There are reports that pectin's were given to children after the Chernobyl disaster in Ukraine. Whilst Teddy didn't ever have radiation treatment, he did have the occasional X-ray and CT scan. Given that my number one rule with supplements is to aim for a product in a natural food type form, on initial review it looks unlikely to cause any harm. At best, if the claims are true, it could help remove some of the aftereffects of radiation from the body. At worst, it's just a good source of dietary fibre as apple pectin's are simply the natural substance found in the cell walls of apples.

Eighteen months after the end of treatment was the time I really started to deep dive into various types of practices to support the body's balance, such as red-light therapy and grounding sheets, which I have written about in other chapters. I also started to work with different types of herbalists with more of a detox specialism, whereas Dr Kate focuses on oncology. We still see Dr Kate today, though, to make sure all of the protocol I have pulled together is meaningful and safe. Now that we see our hospital team so much less, having a qualified doctor who's still on the General Medical Council's register feels reassuring as I have someone to soundboard my ideas with and Dr Kate is willing to listen.

We are also currently going through further testing with Ted by way of hair and stool samples to see what the potential post-treatment impacts are of heavy metals still within the body or gut microbiome deficiencies. This has required a bit more of a financial investment than most of the supplements we use. However, I think we have opted to do it at the right time now that Teddy's body has had significant time to recover and do its best work, whilst supported adequately.

I hope this chapter has given you some food for thought about how you could serve your body so it can do its best work to stay as strong as possible.

CHAPTER 13

LIFE BEYOND THE BELL

"Yesterday is history, tomorrow is a mystery, and today is a gift of the present"

- Bil Keane

This is probably not the fairy tale ending you want to see this book end on, but for us, this is our happy ending. Our son is medically healthy, and he is here with us against all the statistics placed against him. Becoming comfortable with being uncomfortable and accepting that life will never be the same again is the hardest practical lesson that any cancer survivor and their family will ever learn.

At the time of writing this chapter, we are experiencing more challenges. I tell you this not to upset you and tear away hopes of riding into the sunset with cancer in the rear-view mirror but to give you an honest perception of what life really is like after you ring that bell. In six days, it will be two years since Teddy was diagnosed. Teddy has just spent a night in hospital due to catching Flu A and a secondary chest infection. We have been through one of the worst winters for the NHS our consultant has ever seen. Nursery wants to put Ted on special educational needs register due to being developmentally behind his peers, which I fought tooth and nail against. I think it's fair to say things have been pretty rough.

The world wants us to carry on as if our treatments are done, this course is run, and we are on our way back to normal where the past isn't talked about and where everyone pretends that a life-threatening event didn't just occur. Because that would be too scary and too painful and uncomfortable for most people to know what to do or say.

It is here that trauma finally shows up for many, having been kept suppressed by the need to fight.

I don't know exactly what caused my trauma to come out of the cave like a wild lion with its huge fangs on show, ready to destroy anything in its path. It was about two months after Ted's first stem cell transplant anniversary. In my world, we call it the first re-birthday. Teddy had his final line removed, the last physical reminder of treatment. I mustered the courage for the first time to ask our team what the prognosis looked like for Ted and was told we were now looking at ninety-seven percent probability of cure. I had recruited mums across the country to hold stem cell donor drives and we had been featured in major newspapers. Ted and I even went on BBC Breakfast TV (what an honour) to promote our drive and grow the donor register. That weekend the mums and I grew the register by 3500 people with nine hundred signing up within fifteen minutes of Ted and me being on TV. We even found several lifesaving matches;

life was on what felt such a high. But that's what happens when the body relaxes: those feelings start to bubble to the top. They look for a place they feel safe and look for things to worry about.

Whilst you are in treatment, there's always a next step and a weird feeling of hope because there's another treatment planned ahead. Being out of treatment is so much harder because you are scared of what could come next and what your options would be. I was told it would be hard, but you can't really prepare yourself. Life is just different; *you* are different, and I think, in part, surviving the new normal is accepting that when you have a bad day it's ok to want to open the wine or cry on the phone with a friend and that this too shall hopefully pass. Just enjoy the good moments where you can and protect yourself when you need it. For me, this meant muting but not unfollowing other families I was connected with on social media or even deleting the app for a few days when my mental health wasn't good, or Teddy had a virus.

But there have been so many amazing moments as well. Moments when I suddenly realised that I forgot for a minute the pain and suffering we have been through. I often found myself in those early days post-transplant, when Ted's hair started coming back in thick and fast, thinking, "Did that really actually happen to us, or did I imagine it all?"

Winter is proving to be the hardest season. For my family and others, I speak to it's that time between early January and the end of March, but this really depends on where you live. It is the time when the respiratory virus seems to give no let-up, every cough and sniffle fills your body with complete dread, and your mood is low till things have picked up again. There is the constant tilt of the worry seesaw, wondering if this is the sign of a relapse or if this winter bug will now cause a relapse. I actually got very close to pulling the boys out of nursery. The whole situation was a huge trigger for my PTSD. I could make no plans and was angry with the world for going round spreading their germs and plugging their children with Calpol and sending them to school just so their own lives were not inconvenienced.

Going through therapy wasn't something I could consider until at least a year post-transplant when we could breathe that first baby sigh of relief. In fact, it was Ted's clinical nurse specialist – who is equivalent to a medical social worker in the transplant world – who encouraged it. She could see I was really struggling. I would burst into tears at the smallest thing, and we had to have some rules about voicemails as I would completely spiral if I missed her call and then couldn't reach her. She now knows I need her to start the conversation or voicemail off with, "Nothing's wrong," but even then, my mind's not able to be present till I have been able to make contact.

Talking therapy didn't do much for me, even with a psychologist from our hospital who specialises in children's cancer. For me, no amount of talking in this world could undo what we had been through, and my brain had chosen to protect itself by refusing to accept any narrative other than Ted would be ok, he would make it. That's still the case now. However, we were one of the lucky families. Teddy never went to intensive care or high dependency and his body always responded well to treatment, largely due to how we supported him nutritionally.

One thing that has worked really well for me is hypnotherapy, and not the 'I'm going to make you think you are a chicken' type. Hypnotherapy is all about helping your brain get out of flight or flight mode and into a more logical way of thinking. You see, the brain goes back to a place where it feels safe. Not where *you* feel safe but where *it* feels safe. When you have been through trauma, especially the type that blindsides you, it's more comfortable for the brain to go back to that place that fears the most catastrophic of scenarios than a logical one that's actually more likely.

That doesn't stop me living my life on high alert. Maybe I would have always been that kind of mum; I am a natural worrier. That's what led us to a super early diagnosis of only three percent leukaemia in the blood. Google can be my best friend or my worst enemy. Every bruise from normal toddler play gets photographed and analysed in the days that follow. Five minutes before sitting down to write this chapter, I was googling, 'What's a normal number of hairs to find on your pillow?' having put Ted to bed and noticed some loose hairs. (You lose between fifty and one hundred strands a day; in case you are interested.)

I think the bottom line for me is that whilst my child is happy, smiling and full of beans, I am happy, and I can cope. Every day that passes is a day closer to cure. Our lives have been changed forever and in the most horrific of ways, but we are healthier as a family than we would have ever been without cancer, and I go to bed every night with complete gratitude in my heart. The things I have learned about keeping the body strong and fuelling it in the right way are now part of our core beliefs and aren't something I am willing to compromise on for anyone. Whilst some may feel I should relax more and let the children eat more junk, it's fundamentally not a part of my belief system and, frankly, also not how I grew up as a 1980s born child.

The risk of secondary cancer for survivors outside of relapse is there and it's not a chance I'm willing to take. My insurance policy and the way I talk myself off a ledge when times are bad is to remind myself how much we are doing and how well that has served us in the past. Whilst that's without judgement of those who choose a different path, I truly believe that everything you eat, and your environment will either help you or it will harm you. Everything in the universe has a polar opposite: life and death, black and white, ying and yang, sickness and health. With the statistic that one in two of us will get cancer in our lifetime, I refuse to sit back and let that happen to my family again, although I should probably look after my own health a little better and fill my own cup more. Maybe I will start tomorrow.

If I can give you one piece of advice as I conclude this book, it is this.

This method of keeping your body strong is hard, it is exhausting, but it is worth it. At best it could possibly lead to a better outcome and at worst it could help make it a little more bearable and a little easier on the body. Do not be afraid to ask for help and don't be a martyr to feel you have to do it on your own. Being brave and strong in part is about accepting help. I didn't do it on my own; I had a village who were willing to support me and who backed me. People were happy to cook meals to my recipes, to help with our dog and to would take George out on great adventures so he wouldn't suffer too much and to try and distract him from being separated from either parent.

Speaking of George, I think it's important to recognise the trauma he went through even though he appeared to cope well. Nine months post-transplant, I had to take Teddy to hospital in the middle of night with a fever as per transplant rules. George cried hysterically on Facetime the next morning, which led me down the path of understanding about children's developmental trauma. This was a term I reserved until recently for adopted and neglected children. More studies are coming out about the impact of trauma on children under the age of five of medically complex patients or siblings. If ignored, many will be misdiagnosed as being on the spectrum later. At the time, we thought George was managing well but on reflection he was simply masking his anxiety in order to cope with the lack of stability around him. We did our very best and he always had a loving parent around but being separated from his twin has had a lasting effect on him and we are working on this with the help of professionals. Beacon House is a great resource if this could be impacting your family.

I hope this book has given you hope on the journey you find yourself taking. I hope it has allowed you to see that taking control over cancer does have its place and it doesn't have to mean shunning Western medicine. The evidence is there of the power of healing through plants and food, you just need to look in the right places to find it. In the two years I have been on this journey, I started out arguing with medics about the immune system sitting mainly within the gut microbiome to now having these conversations initiated by professionals who are seeing more clinical studies that back what I have always said to them.

I have been as raw and vulnerable as I can be with you, sharing all my best advice because I simply want to see more people survive. I want all of the pain and the hard work we went through not to be in vain, although really, it's never in vain because my beautiful child is here today. I just hope that the things I am teaching him now go on to serve him a long time after I am gone and create lifelong healthy habits because our health is our wealth.

I want to dedicate this book firstly to my husband, Kurt. Bubs, we certainly aren't your traditional lovey-dovey married couple and more has been sent to break us than to keep us together, but we are the ultimate team. Nothing and no one will ever undo our bond, no matter where we end up. I'm so grateful for every time you went into battle for me and helped me get what I needed to help our son. Even though the approach was sometimes a little bullish, I know you would do anything for your family. I don't tell you enough but THANK YOU. I wouldn't have got through this without you.

George, our little firecracker, I hope soon you will know that we are all back to stay. Everything is going to be ok now. I'm sorry I left you more than I wanted to, and I was always thinking of you. I know your heart and I want you to know it wasn't anything you did. We had no choice. I can't imagine what your little heart went through to be separated not only from your mummy but also from your twin at such a young age, the person whose side you had never left since conception. You have been so brave for such a young child. I am in awe of how you handled it even when you were silently struggling. But it's over now, you can relax. I promise I won't leave you again.

And Teddy, the star of the show, as your daddy always said. I can't wait to see you hit more of your milestones and live the life that you deserve more than anyone I know. I wish you were old enough so I can tell you how truly proud I am that you chose me to be your mum, how incredible you are, and the sheer joy you bring when you enter the room. I wish I could make you see how strong you have been, but at the same time I hope you never remember this time and you live a life of ignorance of what cancer really put you through. Reach for the stars, Baroo, no one cares if you land on the moon. Just try not to give me a heart attack too much as you grow up navigating life: grey hairs I can handle, a heart attack not so much. Our time with hospitals is done.

Thank you for reading and I hope you found hope in this book for a brighter future.

Please feel free to reach for additional support:
cancerisntallaboutchemo.com

ABOUT THE AUTHOR

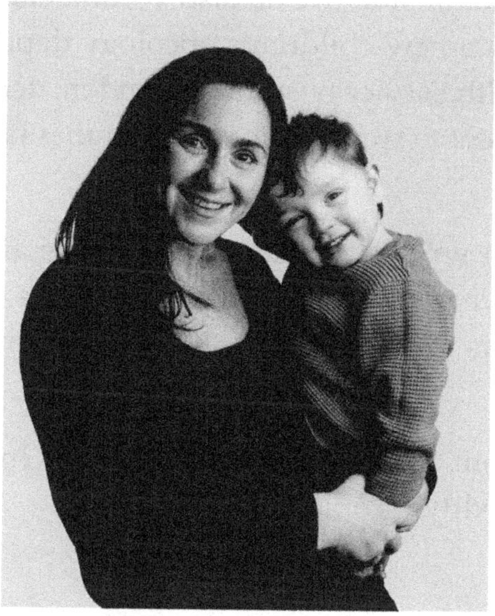

Sarah Cripps is a determined and committed advocate for better nutrition and holistic practices alongside conventional treatment for oncology patients.

She is passionate about integrative nutrition and lifestyle medicine with her story having been featured in the Children's Cancer and Leukaemia Group's award-winning Contact magazine.

After her seventeen-month-old son was diagnosed with Acute Myeloid Leukaemia in April 2022, Sarah drew on her industry experience in nutrition which she has acquired since 2016, in an attempt to help save her son's life.

In 2024 she led a national campaign to grow the UKs national stem cell donor register which received national tv and press coverage and resulted in thousands of new potential donors being registered and a handful of potential genetic matches being identified for people for a donor for a lifesaving bone marrow transplant. She also volunteers her time to help establish a new children's oncology department at a National Health Service hospital in London, demonstrating her commitment to supporting other families facing similar challenges.

Outside of her writing, Sarah enjoys cooking and is known for her creative approach to hiding nutritious foods in her family's meals which she openly shares with her online community.

For more from Sarah please visit her on Instagram or Facebook @Teddys_Tonic

BONUS CHAPTER

FURTHER READING AND REFERENCES

My aim with this book has always been to provide credible evidence for how holistic therapies and approaches, alongside conventional treatment, can potentially improve patient outcomes or reduce the risk of a diagnosis.

The strategies I applied in an attempt to save my son's life came from solid meticulous scientific research, not just blogs or other people's personal accounts.

Whilst some of the advice and treatment recommendations may have been given to me by some of the world's best holistic practitioners, I didn't take their words to be gospel. I still did my research. I don't believe you should ever take anyone's word to be gospel and that includes those who wear white coats.

My ultimate wish for you is that you are able to make informed decisions and have a sense of control over your health.

You will find below a number of resources which I referenced in this book. I have broken them down by chapter to make it easier for you to revisit them. Some of these resources are very scientific and at times the language used in them can be very jargon heavy. This might lead you to feel a little overwhelmed. I know that because that's how I felt at the beginning. I had to learn how to read the studies. I often searched for the meanings of the terminology online. It took time and practice, but it did get easier.

However, for this book to be taken seriously by an oncologist and for a person in active treatment to be able to use it to push their team for the things they want to happen, I have to reference credible scientific sources. This is about the bigger picture and pushing the needle in a way that is more difficult for traditional medicine to dismiss.

There are online tools you can use to translate some of the information into layman's English. I still use these today when I am time poor or feeling tired. In such circumstances I suggest you focus on the abstract and the conclusions sections of the papers to gain a good overview.

Try not to focus too much on the specifics of the cancer types used in trials as this could lead to further overwhelm. I did research Acute Myeloid Leukaemia, of course, but I didn't completely discount research that talked about a different blood cancer such as Acute Lymphoblastic Leukaemia when it came to holistic p. They are both blood cancers. Moreover, cancer all starts with the malfunction of a cell.

Research and trials can sometimes require as few as twenty people who share some predefined characteristics such as the same type of cancer and stage of disease. This can shrink the pool of available people to study. You will need to apply logic based on the hypothesis of the research and regarding the potential benefits versus the risk.

If you want to research further on your own, I highly recommend you first start with the National Institute of Health website (NIH), which you can find at **www.nih.gov** and also PubMed, which can be found at **https://pubmed.ncbi.nlm.nih.gov/**

They are linked but separate entities. The NIH is a part of the U.S. Department of Health and Human Services. It is a government agency that focuses on health and medical research. They fund studies and provide health-related info.

PubMed, on the other hand, is a free online database run by the NIH that offers access to millions of articles and abstracts on health and biomedical topics. It helps people find scientific research easily.

So, NIH is all about research, while PubMed is where you go to find scientific articles and studies about health and medicine.

Please note, if you are reading this book as a paperback rather than an eBook, you can visit my website **www.cancerisntallaboutchemo.com** where you can find all of the resources listed below in a clickable format.

Chapter 1 - Introduction

Title: The Microbiome and Immune Regulation After Transplantation
Find it here: **https://pubmed.ncbi.nlm.nih.gov/27517729/**
PubMed ID: 27517729

Title: The Role of Microbiota in Allogeneic Hematopoietic Stem Cell Transplantation
Find it here: **https://pubmed.ncbi.nlm.nih.gov/33412949/**
PubMed ID: 33412949

Title: Sepsis and the Microbiome: A Vicious Cycle
Find it here: **https://academic.oup.com/jid/article/223/Supplement_3/S264/6039543**
PubMed ID: 33330900

Title: Microbiota as Predictor of Mortality in Allogeneic Hematopoietic-Cell Transplantation
Find it here: **https://pubmed.ncbi.nlm.nih.gov/32101664/**
PubMed ID: 32101664

Title: The Impact of Gut Microbial Signals on Hematopoietic Stem Cells and the Bone Marrow Microenvironment
Find it here: Frontiersin.org, **https://www.frontiersin.org/journals/immunology/articles/10.3389/fimmu.2024.1338178/full**

Title: The Influence of the Gut Microbiome on Cancer, Immunity, and Cancer Immunotherapy
Find it here: NIH, **https://pmc.ncbi.nlm.nih.gov/articles/PMC6529202**

Title: Fibre Fueled: The Plant-Based Gut Health Program for Losing Weight, Restoring Your Health, and Optimizing Your Microbiome, by Dr Will Bulsiewicz
Find it here: Amazon, **https://amzn.to/3AcwRgg**

Title: Dr Will Bulsiewcz on the Microbiome: Heal Your Gut, Sidestep Disease and Thrive
Find it here: YouTube, Rick Roll Podcast, **https://www.youtube.com/watch?v=9jDsQU1UEAo&t=550s**

Title: Diverse Gut Microbiome May Help Children Survive Stem Cell Transplant
Find it here: News Medical, **https://www.news-medical.net/news/20230810/Diverse-gut-microbiome-may-help-children-survive-stem-cell-transplant.aspx**

Chapter 2 - Can We Control the Cause of Cancer?

Title: The Cancer Prevention, Anti-Inflammatory and Anti-Oxidation of Bioactive Phytochemicals Targeting the TLR4 Signalling Pathway
Find it here: **https://www.mdpi.com/1422-0067/19/9/2729**

Title: Epigenetic Contribution to Cancer
Find it here: **https://www.sciencedirect.com/science/article/abs/pii/S1937644824000881?via%3Dihub**
Pubmed ID: 39179345

Title: Epigenetics/Epigenomics and Prevention of Early Stages of Cancer by Isothiocyanates Review
Find it here: **https://pmc.ncbi.nlm.nih.gov/articles/PMC8044264/**
Pubmed ID: 33055265

Title: Dietary Epigenetics in Cancer and Aging
Find it here: **https://pmc.ncbi.nlm.nih.gov/articles/PMC3875399/**
Pubmed ID: 24114485

Title: Targeting Epigenetic Regulators for Cancer Therapy: Mechanisms and Advances in Clinical Trials
Find it here: **https://pmc.ncbi.nlm.nih.gov/articles/PMC6915746/**
Pubmed ID: PMC6915746

Title: Dirty Genes, by Dr Ben Lynch
Find it here: Amazon, **https://amzn.to/3ZcZLFE**

Title: Cancer as a Metabolic Disease: On the Origin, Management, and Prevention of Cancer, by Thomas Seyfried
Find it here: Amazon, **https://amzn.to/4i3QvMw**

Chapter 3 - Diet

Title: American Gut: An Open Platform for Citizen Science Microbiome Research
Find it here: **https://pubmed.ncbi.nlm.nih.gov/29795809/**
Pubmed ID: 29795809

Title: Achieving Longevity Through Your Favorite Foods
Find it here: Dr WilliamLi.com, **https://drwilliamli.com/achieving-longevity-through-your-favorite-foods/**

Title: Eat To Beat Disease, by Dr William Li
Find it here: Amazon, **https://amzn.to/3CIewbP**

Title: Angiogenesis Inhibitors
Find it here: National Cancer Institute, **https://www.cancer.gov/about-cancer/treatment/types/immunotherapy/angiogenesis-inhibitors-fact-sheet**

Title: Can We Eat to Starve Cancer
Find it here: YouTube, **https://www.youtube.com/watch?v=OjkzfeJz66o&t=100s**

Title: 10% Human: How Your Body's Microbes Hold the Key to Health and Happiness, by Alanna Collen
Find it here: Amazon, **https://amzn.eu/d/e6Vt0lV**

Title: The Interplay Between the Gut Microbiome and the Immune System in the Context of Infectious Diseases Throughout Life and the Role of Nutrition in Optimizing Treatment Strategies
Find it here: **https://pubmed.ncbi.nlm.nih.gov/33803407/**
Pubmed ID: 33803407

Title: Prebiotics: Ignored Player in the Fight Against Cancer
Find it here: **https://pmc.ncbi.nlm.nih.gov/articles/PMC10644333/**

Title: Therapeutic Effect of Blueberry Extracts for Acute Myeloid Leukaemia
Find it here: **https://pmc.ncbi.nlm.nih.gov/articles/PMC5875929/**
Pubmed ID: 29607443

Title: Is There a Role for Carbohydrate Restriction in the Treatment and Prevention of Cancer?
Find it here: **https://pmc.ncbi.nlm.nih.gov/articles/PMC3267662/**

Chapter 4 - Supplements

Natural Medicines Database - For drug and supplement contraindications
https://naturalmedicines.therapeuticresearch.com/

Title: Regulation of Cell Cycle Transition and Induction of Apoptosis in HL-60 Leukaemia Cells by the Combination of Coriolus Versicolor and Ganoderma Lucidum
Find it here: **https://pubmed.ncbi.nlm.nih.gov/23670292/**
Pubmed ID: 23670292

Title: Cordyceps Militaris Exerts Anticancer Effect on Non–Small Cell Lung Cancer by Inhibiting Hedgehog Signalling via Suppression of TCTN3
Find it here: **https://pmc.ncbi.nlm.nih.gov/articles/PMC7265736/**
Pubmed ID: 32456485

Title: Hericium Erinaceus (Lion's Mane) Mushroom Extracts Inhibit Metastasis of Cancer Cells to the Lung in CT-26 Colon Cancer-transplanted Mice
Find it here: **https://pubmed.ncbi.nlm.nih.gov/23668749/**
Pubmed ID: 23668749

Title: Chaga Mushroom Extract Suppresses Oral Cancer Cell Growth via Inhibition of Energy Metabolism
Find it here: **https://pubmed.ncbi.nlm.nih.gov/38720012/**
Pubmed ID: 38720012

Title: Phase 1 Clinical Trial of Trametes Versicolor in Women With Breast Cancer
Find it here: **https://pubmed.ncbi.nlm.nih.gov/22701186/**
Pubmed ID: 22701186

Chapter 6 - Stress

Title: Meditation Programs for Psychological Stress and Well-being: A Systematic Review and Meta-analysis
Find it here: **https://pmc.ncbi.nlm.nih.gov/articles/PMC4142584/**

Title: The Benefits of Mindfulness in Mental Healthcare Professionals
Find it here: **https://pmc.ncbi.nlm.nih.gov/articles/PMC8943343/**

Title: Chronic Stress Promotes Cancer Development
Find it here: **https://pmc.ncbi.nlm.nih.gov/articles/PMC7466429/**

Title: Interplay Between Stress and Cancer—A Focus on Inflammation
Find it here: **https://pmc.ncbi.nlm.nih.gov/articles/PMC10067747/**
Pubmed ID: 37020461

Title: Association of Stress-Related Disorders With Subsequent Autoimmune Disease
Find it here: **https://jamanetwork.com/journals/jama/fullarticle/2685155**

Title: New Uses of Hypnosis in the Treatment of Posttraumatic Stress Disorder
Find it here: **https://pubmed.ncbi.nlm.nih.gov/2211565/**
Pubmed ID: 2211565

Chapter 8 - Complementary Therapies

Title: Healing the Gerson Way, by Charlotte Gersen
Find it here: Amazon, **https://amzn.to/3V9LIiD**

Fasting

Title: Fast Like a Girl, by Dr Mindy Peltz
Find it here: Amazon, **https://amzn.to/4i6DSjD**

Title: To Fast, or Not to Fast Before Chemotherapy, That Is the Question
Find it here: **https://pmc.ncbi.nlm.nih.gov/articles/PMC5870384/**
Pubmed ID: 29587670

Title: Changes in Human Gut Microbiota Composition Are Linked to the Energy Metabolic Switch During 10 d of Buchinger Fasting
Find it here: Cambridge.org, **https://www.cambridge.org/core/journals/journal-of-nutritional-science/article/changes-in-human-gut-microbiota-composition-are-linked-to-the-energy-metabolic-switch-during-10-d-of-buchinger-fasting/1E4307FAFD57B566BE13193A09037673**

Title: Prolonged Nightly Fasting and Breast Cancer Prognosis
Find it here: **https://jamanetwork.com/journals/jamaoncology/fullarticle/2506710**

Title: When Fasting Gets Tough, the Tough Immune Cells Get Going—or Die
Find it here: **https://pmc.ncbi.nlm.nih.gov/articles/PMC7474734/**

Title: Fasting-like Diet Turns the Immune System Against Cancer
Find it here: USC Today, **https://today.usc.edu/fasting-like-diet-turns-the-immune-system-against-cancer/**

Grounding

Title: Grounding – The Universal Anti-inflammatory Remedy
Find it here: **https://pmc.ncbi.nlm.nih.gov/articles/PMC10105021/**
Pubmed ID: 36528336

Title: The Effects of Grounding (Earthing) on Inflammation, the Immune Response, Wound Healing, and Prevention and Treatment of Chronic Inflammatory and Autoimmune Diseases
Find it here: **https://pmc.ncbi.nlm.nih.gov/articles/PMC4378297/**
Pubmed ID: 25848315

Title: Earthing and Grounding in Cancer Care: A Holistic Approach
Find it here: Cancer for Healing,
https://cancercenterforhealing.com/earthing-and-grounding-in-cancer-care/

Title: The Earthing Movie: The Remarkable Science of Grounding (full documentary)
Find it here: Online Streaming Sites, YouTube, **https://www.youtube.com/watch?v=44ddtR0XDVU&t=200s**

Homoeopathy

Title: Is There Good Scientific Evidence for Homeopathy?
Find it here: **https://www.takingcharge.csh.umn.edu/there-good-scientific-evidence-homeopathy**

Title: Is There a Role for Homeopathy in Cancer Care? Questions and Challenges
Find it here: **https://pubmed.ncbi.nlm.nih.gov/26210222/**
Pubmed ID: 26210222

Title: Perceptions of Homeopathy in Supportive Cancer Care Among Oncologists and General Practitioners in France
Find it here: **https://pubmed.ncbi.nlm.nih.gov/33763723/**
Hyperbaric Oxygen Therapy

Title: Hyperbaric Oxygen Therapy and Cancer–a review
Find it here: **https://pubmed.ncbi.nlm.nih.gov/23054400/**

Title: Hyperbaric Oxygen Therapy Adjuvant Chemotherapy and Radiotherapy Through Inhibiting Stemness in Glioblastoma
Find it here: **https://pubmed.ncbi.nlm.nih.gov/37886967/**

Title: Effect of Hyperbaric Oxygen on the Anticancer Effect of Artemisinin on Molt-4 Human Leukaemia Cells
Find it here: **https://pubmed.ncbi.nlm.nih.gov/21115894/**
Pubmed ID: 21115894

Title: Advances in Hyperbaric Oxygen to Promote Immunotherapy Through Modulation of the Tumour Microenvironment
Find it here: **https://pmc.ncbi.nlm.nih.gov/articles/PMC10543083/**

Title: Can HBOT Help Fight Cancer?
Find it here: YouTube, HBOT USA, **https://www.youtube.com/watch?v=n8XRPQyuXSg**

Title: Hyperbaric Oxygen Therapy Counters Oxidative Stress/Inflammation-Driven Symptoms in Long COVID-19 Patients
Find it here: **https://pmc.ncbi.nlm.nih.gov/articles/PMC10608857/**
Pubmed ID: 37887357
Near Infra-Red Light Therapy

Title: Effects of Low-Level Laser Therapy in the Healing of Oral Mucositis Induced by Chemotherapy
Find it here: **https://pubmed.ncbi.nlm.nih.gov/31360381/**
Pubmed ID: 31360381

Title: Photobiomodulation Therapy in Management of Cancer Therapy-induced Side Effects: WALT position paper 2022
Find it here: **https://pubmed.ncbi.nlm.nih.gov/36110957/**
Pubmed ID: 36110957

Title: Photobiomodulation for the Treatment of Acute and Chronic Pain
Find it here: Science Direct.com, **https://www.sciencedirect.com/science/article/abs/pii/S1011134419303227**

Reiki

Title: What Does the Evidence Say About Reiki for Cancer?
Find it here: Ons.org, **https://www.ons.org/publications-research/voice/news-views/what-does-evidence-say-about-reiki-cancer**

Title: Reiki Is Better Than Placebo and Has Broad Potential as a Complementary Health Therapy
Find it here: **https://journals.sagepub.com/doi/full/10.1177/2156587217728644**

Chapter 9 - Question Everything

Title: Infection Control Manual – Section 5 Food and Beverages
Find it here: **https://www.nhsborders.scot.nhs.uk/media/127534/internet-use-only-5-food-and-beverage.pdf**

Title: Food Safety for People Having chemotherapy (Systemic Anti-Cancer Treatment)
Find it here: **https://www.buckshealthcare.nhs.uk/pifs/food-safety-for-people-having-chemotherapy/**

Chapter 10 - PEG and NG Tube Feeding

Tube Feeding
Title: Systematic Review of Gastrostomy Complications and Outcomes in Paediatric Cancer and Bone Marrow Transplant
Find it here: **https://pubmed.ncbi.nlm.nih.gov/34245471/**
Pubmed ID: 34245471

Chapter 11 - Teddy's Plan Exactly as We Did it

Title: Cancer Inhibition by Inositol Hexaphosphate (IP6) and Inositol: From Laboratory to Clinic
Find it here: **https://www.sciencedirect.com/science/article/pii/S002231662302535X?via%3Dihub**
Pubmed ID: 14608114

Title: Protection Against Cancer by Dietary IP6 and Inositol
Find it here: **https://pubmed.ncbi.nlm.nih.gov/17044765/**
Pubmed ID: 17044765

Title: Effect of Inositol hexaphosphate (IP(6)) on human normal and leukaemic haematopoietic cells
Find it here: **https://pubmed.ncbi.nlm.nih.gov/12028025/**
Pubmed ID: 12028025

Title: Therapeutic Effect of Blueberry Extracts for Acute Myeloid Leukaemia
Find it here: **https://pubmed.ncbi.nlm.nih.gov/29607443/**
Pubmed ID: 12028025

Title: Investigating Anti-cancer Activity of Dual-loaded Liposomes With Thymoquinone and Vitamin C
Find it here: **https://pubmed.ncbi.nlm.nih.gov/38449422/**
Pubmed ID: 38449422

Title: The role of Coenzyme Q10 as a Preventive and Therapeutic Agent for the Treatment of Cancers
Find it here: **https://pubmed.ncbi.nlm.nih.gov/38330781/**
Pubmed ID: 38330781

Title: Vitamin D Regulates Microbiome-dependent Cancer Immunity
Find it here: **https://pmc.ncbi.nlm.nih.gov/articles/PMC7615937/**
Pubmed ID: **38662827**

Chapter 12 - Detox

Title: Bristol Stool Form Chart
Find it here: Stanford.Edu, **https://pediatricsurgery.stanford.edu/Conditions/BowelManagement/bristol-stool-form-scale.html**

Title: Treating a Herxheimer Reaction With Integrative Medicine
Find it here: Rupa Health.com, **https://www.rupahealth.com/post/treating-a-herxheimer-reaction-with-integrative-medicine**

Title: Excretion of Ni, Pb, Cu, As, and Hg in Sweat Under Two Sweating Conditions
Find it here: **https://pubmed.ncbi.nlm.nih.gov/35410004/**
Pubmed ID: 35410004

Made in the USA
Monee, IL
19 August 2026

60466055R20118